W9-BUO-886

An Invitation to Personal Change

An Invitation to Personal Change

Dianne Hales, M.S. | Kenneth W. Christian, Ph.D.

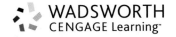

WADSWORTH
CENGAGE Learning

Australia • Brazil • Japan • Korea • Mexico • Singapore • Spain • United Kingdom • United States

WADSWORTH
CENGAGE Learning

An Invitation to Personal Change
Dianne Hales, Kenneth W. Christian

Development Editor: Anna Lustig

Assistant Editor: Elesha Feldman

Editorial Assistant: Sarah Farrant

Technology Project Manager: Lauren Tarson

Marketing Assistant: Katherine Malatesta

Marketing Communications Manager:
  Belinda Krohmer

Project Manager, Editorial Production:
  Trudy Brown

Creative Director: Rob Hugel

Art Director: John Walker

Print Buyer: Paula Vang

Permissions Editor: Bob Kauser

Production Service: Graphic World Inc.

Text Designer: Jeanne Calabrese

Cover Designer: Bill Stanton

Cover Image: Beth Dixson/Alamy

Compositor: Graphic World Inc.

© 2009 Wadsworth, Cengage Learning

ALL RIGHTS RESERVED. No part of this work covered by the copyright herein may be reproduced, transmitted, stored, or used in any form or by any means, graphic, electronic, or mechanical, including but not limited to photocopying, recording, scanning, digitizing, taping, Web distribution, information networks, or information storage and retrieval systems, except as permitted under Section 107 or 108 of the 1976 United States Copyright Act, without the prior written permission of the publisher.

For product information and technology assistance, contact us at
Cengage Learning Customer & Sales Support, 1-800-354-9706
For permission to use material from this text or product,
submit all requests online at **cengage.com/permissions**
Further permissions questions can be e-mailed to
permissionrequest@cengage.com

Library of Congress Control Number: 2008922444

ISBN-13: 978-0-495-39017-6

ISBN-10: 0-495-39017-8

Wadsworth
10 Davis Drive
Belmont, CA 94002-3098
USA

Cengage Learning is a leading provider of customized learning solutions with office locations around the globe, including Singapore, the United Kingdom, Australia, Mexico, Brazil, and Japan. Locate your local office at **international.cengage.com/region**

Cengage Learning products are represented in Canada by Nelson Education, Ltd.

For your course and learning solutions, visit **academic.cengage.com**

Purchase any of our products at your local college store or at our preferred online store **www.ichapters.com**

Printed in Canada
1 2 3 4 5 6 7 12 11 10 09 08

CONTENTS

v

TO THE INSTRUCTOR

We are offering you an invitation that your students will not want to turn down. *An Invitation to Personal Change* (IPC), unlike any other textbook, supplement, or manual, does not merely talk about personal change. Based on decades of psychological research and clinical practice, IPC serves as a curriculum for change, inviting students to take appropriate action in simple, compellingly straightforward ways. Its groundbreaking labs present step-by-step blueprints for creating healthier habits, eliminating harmful behaviors, maximizing performance, and achieving greater physical, psychological, and spiritual well-being.

An Invitation to Personal Change, designed for use as either an ancillary or a standalone text, grew out of our lifelong commitment to helping people achieve their greatest potential. One of us, Dianne Hales is the author of the top-selling *Invitation to Health* textbooks, acclaimed for their engaging, student-friendly style and sound scientific basis. The other, Dr. Kenneth W. Christian, a psychologist with extensive experience in both academics and clinical practice, founded the Maximum Potential Project in 1990 to study and foster personal achievement and fulfillment. In IPC, we have honed and targeted a tested, evidence-based approach to personal change for college students.

The structure of this book and its labs moves students through the changes of stage postulated by psychologist James Prochaska and his colleagues—from what Prochaska refers to as precontemplation all the way through to action and the maintenance of new habits. Other major sources include Milton Erickson's emphasis on the role of indirect suggestion in change, Albert Ellis's rational-emotive therapy, the cognitive behavioral movement, Martin Seligman's work on positive psychology, James Pennebaker's studies of the power of journaling, contemporary neuroscience research on the plasticity of the brain, and the social psychology research of Shelly Taylor and many, many others.

Rather than simply presenting the insights into personal change of these researchers and practitioners, we have translated theory and research into practical "power tools" that empower students to direct change in their lives. Our labs take students through the stages of change, following a uniform structure that can serve as a template for future changes as well. By making immediate practical changes, they learn the fundamental steps involved in any future change.

Why a Book on Personal Change?

Of all the lessons you teach your students, none may be more enduring or valuable than how to personally direct change in their lives. Regardless of their age, socioeconomic status, ethnic background, or life circumstances, your students are facing challenges and change every day. The choices they make, and the ways they respond now, shape their futures and their lives.

The stakes are high. As you know, college can be a time of experimentation and risk taking. Four in ten undergraduates are binge drinkers; one in four smokes. Among those who are sexually active, almost three in four say they have engaged in unprotected sex. Only about a third of college students exercise regularly. Their nutrition is notoriously poor. Weights—and weight problems—are rising on campus. More students are struggling with stress and seeking psychological counseling. By the time they graduate, one in four students has at least one major risk factor for diabetes, metabolic syndrome, or heart disease.

Yet even those students who want to change their behavior often have no idea how to begin. *An Invitation to Personal Change* fills this gap by equipping students with the practical skills they need both to break unhealthy habits and to make positive changes that enhance their well-being. Ours is not a pop psych, quick-fix, overnight solution but an integrated, carefully constructed program for personal change. Students will be able to use the insights, techniques, and strategies given in this book not just for your course but throughout their lives.

How to Use IPC

An Invitation to Personal Change is a practical handbook for students in a range of courses, including not only health, wellness, fitness, nutrition, health counseling, health psychology, and physical education but also college success, business, and positive psychology. Available in print and electronic form, IPC consists of three elements.

The first element is the main text, which has two parts. The first presents the fundamentals of personal change, including the latest insights from neuroscience, the stages of change, and the basic principles of behavioral change. To make these relevant for students, we have created six vignettes in our "Real Change" features that use personal narratives to illustrate how students in diverse circumstances—incoming freshmen, commuters, immigrants, older students, working students, parents—encounter common dilemmas and use the personal change tools in IPC to analyze their situations and make better choices and healthier changes.

The second part of the main text introduces the practical applications of personal change psychology. Nine chapters, each dedicated to an essential power tool, provide assessments, inventories, goal-setting and journaling exercises, and classroom activities. Some are assignable; others encourage personal and private reflection on values, attitudes, goals, motivations, strengths, dreams, and patterns of thinking and self-talk.

The Labs for An Invitation to Personal Change

The second element is the lab manual. Each lab follows Prochaska's stages of change, which we have renamed "Get Real," "Get Ready," "Get Going," and "Lock It In." Students can use this four-part approach, as we have mentioned, as a template to create their own personal change maps for *any* personal change they want to make.

In "Get Real," students take a realistic audit of where they are so that they can determine where to go. The "Get Ready" section provides instructions and exercises designed to prepare them for making the actual behavioral change, such as identifying and gathering support and resources. "Get Going" involves initiating and beginning to practice new, more effective thoughts and behaviors that will replace old, ineffective, self-defeating ones. "Lock It In" ensures enduring change by teaching students how to deal with setbacks and how to integrate personal change permanently into their lives.

Lab topics are as follows:

- *Psychological and spiritual well-being:* "The Grateful Thread," "Soul Food," "Your Personal Balance Point," "Defusing Test Stress," "Rx: Relax," "Your Psychological Self-Care Pyramid," "Taming a Toxic Temper," "Finity"
- *Healthy habits:* "Excise Exercise Excuses," "Mind over Platter," "Thinking Thinner," "Sleep Power"
- *Behavioral choices:* "Do It Now," "To Have or Have Not," "Don't Go There," "Your Alcohol Audit," "Butt Out," "The Sexiness of Safer Sex"
- *Communication and relationship skills:* "Help Yourself," "Listen Up," "What's Your Intimacy Quotient?"
- *Social dimensions of health:* "Health Assurance," "Your Guardian Angel," "Our-Space"

We recommend that all students complete the one-week introductory lab "Choosing to Change, Choosing a Change" to identify the behavioral changes that are most relevant and compelling for them as they begin the class. We further suggest that students take on no more than two labs at a time, although we believe they will find nearly every lab beneficial over the course of their college life and into the future.

IPC Journal

The third element is the *Journal for An Invitation to Personal Change*. We emphasize journaling—the process of putting feelings and thoughts into written words—as an industrial-strength power tool for personal change. Most of the exercises in IPC and in the labs require students to use this form of expressive writing to reflect; evaluate past, present, and future behavior; and gain insight into their feelings.

To make it as easy and as engaging as possible to develop the journaling habit, we are separately publishing the *IPC Journal* coordinated with the exercises in Part II of IPC and in the lab manual. This notebook makes it easy for students to complete their journaling assignments and helps ensure that they experience journaling as a supportive tool for ongoing personal change and greater self-understanding, one they will use for the rest of their lives.

Who We Are

Dianne Hales, M.S., is one of the most widely published and honored health writers in the country. Her best-selling textbooks include *An Invitation to Health, An Invitation to Health Brief,* and *An Invitation to Wellness.* Her trade books include the award-winning compendium of mental health information, *Caring for the Mind: The Comprehensive Guide to Mental Health; Think Thin, Be Thin* (with Doris Helmering); *Just Like a Woman: How Gender Science Is Redefining What Makes Us Female; The Mind/Mood Pill Book; Intensive Caring: New Hope for High-Risk Pregnancy* (with Dr. Timothy Johnson); *How to Sleep Like a Baby; The U.S. Army Total Fitness Program; New Hope for Problem Pregnancies;* and *The Complete Book of Sleep.*

Dianne also is a contributing editor for *Parade* and has written more than 2,000 articles for national publications. She has received numerous writing awards, including prizes from the American Psychiatric Association, American Psychological Association, National Women's Political Caucus, California Psychiatric Society, Children and Adults with Attention Deficit/Hyperactivity (CHADD), Council for the Advancement of Scientific Education, and New York City Public Library.

Kenneth W. Christian, Ph.D., is the founder and director of the Maximum Potential Project, an innovative research-based program designed to conquer underachievement. His trade book, *Your Own Worst Enemy: Breaking the Habits of Adult Underachievement,* which has been translated and published in Brazil, the People's Republic of China, Russia, Croatia, and Poland, is based on his experience and findings. As cofounder and director for 23 years of the highly regarded Lafayette Therapy Center in the San Francisco Bay Area, he conducted systems interventions, family therapy, and extensive group and individual therapy using solution-focused psychoeducational methods.

Dr. Christian has held faculty positions at the University of California at Davis and Lone Mountain College in San Francisco, where he served for six years as director of the graduate program in clinical psychology. He has taught undergraduate courses in personality theory, social psychology, experimental psychology, and altered states of consciousness. He has extensive experience as a consultant in change management, leadership development, team building, and performance optimization.

Join the IPC Team

Change is built into the DNA of *An Invitation to Personal Change.* We expect it to evolve, zeroing in ever more precisely on your students' needs, goals, and priorities yet extending to more areas of their lives. We invite you to be part of these changes. Please let us know what you think, how the IPC package is working for you and your students, what you like about it, what you would like to see in future versions. We look forward to working with you.

Dianne and Ken
IPC.Authors@gmail.com

TO THE STUDENT

We are inviting you to a place you may never have been: the director's chair. No, you haven't stumbled into a film course. *An Invitation to Personal Change* (IPC, as we call it) proposes a new way of thinking about your life: as a movie, complete with action, drama, plot twists, sets, costumes, and supporting cast. Reading this book, completing its exercises and labs, and using your *Journal for An Invitation to Personal Change* will equip you with the skills you need to direct change—to write the script and call the shots for the story of you.

The single most important and enduring lesson you can learn in college, we contend, is how to make positive personal changes. Whether you are using IPC as a requirement for a class or not, we want to alert you: This could be the book that changes your life by teaching you how to make the changes you want. It shows you, step by step, how to take stock of where you are, focus on where you're heading, and prepare, initiate, carry out, and maintain change.

However old you are, wherever you came from, whatever your goals, change is and will always be the only sure thing in your life. You've been changing since you were born. Every day you continue to change, inside and out. But change doesn't have to just *happen*. By gaining insight and expertise, you create change. There is no magic, no hidden secret to getting the life you want. But there are techniques and tools that, if you use them, empower you to move from where you are at this moment to where you want to be. You will discover and master them here.

You may have thought of personal change as frightening, painful, or even impossible. But now it's time to know the truth: You can direct the changes you want. IPC's approach, based on decades of scientific research and clinical practice, provides simple, compelling, straightforward blueprints for creating healthier habits, eliminating harmful behaviors, and achieving greater physical, psychological, and spiritual well-being. By changing your choices, you change your future and your life. You jump into the director's chair, sit tall and strong, call for action, and take charge of your life—the greatest story you'll ever tell.

Let us hear how it turns out. We welcome any feedback you care to share with us.

Good luck—and enjoy the journey,

Dianne and Ken

IPC.Authors@gmail.com

An Invitation to Personal Change

PART ONE

The New Science of Personal Change

Directing Change

You have been changing since the moment you were born. Every day your body manufactures new cells. Your muscles break down and build up new tissue. Your brain fires new connections. These internal changes occur without any conscious effort on your part.

Each day ushers in other changes, great and small. People come into and go out of your life. Businesses boom and bust. Politicians win and lose elections. Even the global climate changes. These external changes occur whether or not you want or welcome them.

Personal change is different because it is not something that happens to you but is something that *you* do or direct by conscious or nonconscious choice. Anyone can learn how—in the same way that you learn to ride a bike, drive a car, speak Italian, or solve a quadratic equation. Thirty years ago college students wrote papers with type-writers, listened to music on audiocassettes, and mailed letters home. Yes, technology changed, but the people who learned to use computers, MP3 players, and e-mail had to decide to make changes, too.

Our understanding of personal change itself has changed. Thanks to decades of research, we now know what sets the stage for change, how change progresses, and what the keys are to lasting change. We also know that personal change is neither mysterious nor magical but a methodical science that anyone can master.

Simply by being human, you are magnificently equipped for this task. Our species would have died out eons ago if we did not possess remarkable skills for adapting to new challenges and circumstances. You, as the descendent of resourceful, resilient survivors, are hardwired to deal with and initiate change. And change changes you.

Every time you learn something new, whether it's rock climbing or rocket science, you change your possibilities. Whenever you stretch yourself to understand another point of view, you change your range of knowledge. When you tackle a challenging task and dare to fail, you change your capacity to grow. Without such changes you would remain a smaller, paler, narrower shadow of whom and what you can become.

An Invitation to Personal Change poses a fundamental question: Do you choose to change—that is, to continue to develop and move beyond where you are now—or do you tread water and just get by? Let us be clear: We have a definite bias. We come down on the side of making the changes that will allow you to target and achieve your personal goals.

Your other textbooks and courses prepare you for further academic pursuits and a future career. *An Invitation to Personal Change* prepares you for life, which is, in fact, the big school—one continuous opportunity to learn. If personal change were easy, there would be no need for this book. If it were impossible, we wouldn't waste your time or ours trying to convince you otherwise. You—and only you—can make the changes you want happen. *An Invitation to Personal Change* will show you how.

All about Change

We are not discounting the wisdom of great literature or the relevance of world history, but we believe that the single most important lesson you can learn in college is how to direct change. We use the word *direct* deliberately. On a movie set one person calls the shots: the director, who determines when action begins and ends, how many run-throughs and takes the actors must do, which scenes to edit and which to put into the final cut. The director's job is making choices. And that's what personal change is all about.

As the director of your life, you have the power to choose. Remember: Even not choosing is a choice. When you make deliberate choices, you take control—of your time, your health, your relationships, your achievements, and your future. Of course, you cannot control every aspect of your life. All of us enter the world with certain givens, and there is an element of unpredictability to what happens around us. But you have more control over what happens to you than anyone or anything else.

You decide what to eat; whether to drink or smoke; when to study, sleep, and exercise; how to express your sexuality; whether you want to repair or end a friendship. You may not notice the consequences of your choices for months or even years, but their ultimate impact is undeniable.

Don't worry that you're somehow not ready or qualified to sit in the director's chair. You have the capacity and the strength you need. You have only to decide to use them. As you do, keep in mind the following fundamentals:

- **Personal change demands no prerequisites.** You don't have to wait for a burst of insight or a jolt of inspiration. You don't need a guru, coach, or therapist. Change starts with something extremely commonplace: observing what you do *now* and thinking through different choices that might make your life easier, more efficient, or infinitely more satisfying. Once you create this vision, you can prepare your plan for directing change.

- **Personal change is a process.** You don't decide to change one evening and wake up a changed person in the morning. There is no on–off toggle switch, no all-or-nothing experience that clearly divides your life into what was and what will be. You are changing as you read these words because new ideas are entering your brain. Will they lead to lasting change? That depends, again, on your choice. But if you are open, the process of change is already under way. We explain more about the stages of this process later in this chapter.

- **Personal change occurs in steps.** Unless you have been blessed with extraordinary natural talent, you don't sit down at a piano for the first time and play a Beethoven concerto. Instead, you start with the classic five easy pieces. Slowly, steadily, you make progress until one day something seems to click. Suddenly you're making music rather than playing notes. But you've also learned all kinds of other things: how to position your body, use your fingers and hands, recognize rhythm, read notes—so much! When you take small, methodical steps toward a goal, you acquire more than one new competence. If you pay attention, you teach yourself how to direct change.

- **Personal change proceeds better with scientifically tested tools.** Many people change by trial and error. If they want to lose weight, for instance, they try the latest trendy diet—then the next and the next. Unfortunately, the diet yo-yo usually leaves them heavier than ever. But there are powerful research-based tools, which we present in Part II of this book, that dramatically increase the odds of successful change. If you use them consciously and conscientiously, they make change nearly inevitable. Some are as simple as focusing your attention with laserlike intensity or changing the language you use when talking to yourself. These tools, applied consistently, will spare you a lot of wasted time and needless frustration.

- **Personal change replaces old habits with new skills.** You couldn't get through the day without habits. Your daily routine consists of habitual behaviors like combing your hair, getting dressed, taking notes, surfing the web, and a thousand other things. But if you take the time to step back and observe yourself, you may identify some habits that get in your way and slow you down. Maybe you procrastinate, so you're always running behind. Maybe you've never gotten a grip on managing money. Maybe you drink or gamble more than you want. You can replace these negative behaviors with positive new *skills* (the word people use for habits they like and want to keep) that empower and energize your life. The *Labs for An Invitation to Personal Change*, which contains blueprints for personal change, will guide you through the process of making positive change an ongoing part of your life.

■ **Personal change requires time, as well as effort.** To change you must adopt an appropriate long-range perspective. Instead of planning a quick fix, the emotional equivalent of a crash diet, think in terms of revising forever the specific, decisive aspects of your life that will make a difference. People who lose weight and keep it off don't go on—and inevitably off—a diet. They permanently change the way they eat and exercise. The key word is *permanently*. Lasting revisions take time and diligence, although not as much as you might suppose—and not more than you can muster.

Can People Really Change?

Some people make few intentional changes in life. Sure, over time they may get fatter and flabbier, gather lines, and go gray. But they wear their hair the same way, buy the same brand of shoes, eat the same breakfast, and cling to routines for no reason other than the ease of a comfortable, predictable life. Yet as both research and real life show, many others do make important changes. They train for marathons, quit smoking, switch fields, write screenplays, take up the acoustic guitar, or learn to tango even if they never danced before in their lives.

What is the difference between these two groups of people? Their outlook. People who change do not question whether change is possible or look for reasons they cannot change. They simply decide on a change they want and do what is necessary to accomplish it. Changing, which always stems from a resolute decision, becomes job number one. When people do not change, the reason is not that change isn't possible; it's that they put the brakes on change or limit their possibilities by presuming they cannot change and looking for reasons to prove it.

Of course, there are things you can't change. You can't alter when and where you were born. You can't do anything but complain about the weather. You cannot fly regardless of how furiously you flap your arms. But often you think you cannot do something simply because you have never done it before.

Footprints in the Brain

We are born with 23 billion brain cells, or neurons. Each neuron connects to hundreds of other neurons by anywhere from 1,000 to 10,000 synapses. Until quite recently scientists believed that the brain itself could not change and that no new neurons or synapses formed after birth. This theory has been soundly disproved.

The brain and spinal cord contain stem cells, which turn into thousands of new neurons each day. The process of creating new brain cells and synapses occurs most rapidly in childhood but continues throughout life, even into old age. Whenever you learn and change, you establish new neural networks.

Yet we are naturally inclined to stick with the patterns of thinking and acting that we already know. Psychiatrist Milton Erickson, a pioneer in helping people change, told a story from his boyhood to explain how this happens. When he was growing up in Nevada in the early 1900s, he delighted in waking up to a new snowfall. He'd rush to leave for school so that he could be the first to stomp a path through the fresh snow to the local schoolhouse. Often he'd intentionally zig and zag rather than taking the most direct route. Regardless of how circuitous his track, inevitably the next kid would follow it, as would the next, and the next. By the end of the day, the winding route became the one and only path everyone took to school—at least until the snow melted.

This, Erickson contended, is how habits form. We continue to do things the way we always did because we're following a familiar track. Each time we repeat the same sequence of actions, we strengthen these connections. The pathways become so familiar that they are taken automatically, even if they lead nowhere or waste time and energy.

To direct a change—whether it's to eliminate a bad habit or to create a good one—we have to do two things: resist the natural tendency to follow the well-trod path of least resistance and repeat new actions that forge new connections in the brain. For highly elaborate changes such as learning to write with your nondominant hand, this process can be long and arduous. But if you observe yourself closely, you will see that you are already adept at creating simpler habits. In a large lecture hall, you are likely to return to the same seat every day. If you attend church regularly, you head for the same pew. It does not occur to you to stop and consider alternatives. Changing requires you to pay attention to your choices, make new ones, and deliberately repeat the new ones until they become automatic or habitual.

Although venturing into new territory can feel unnerving, the discomfort is temporary. Every time you repeat your new behavior, you strengthen new connections in your brain. If you ever worked with weights, you remember how sore your biceps felt in the beginning. But if you persisted, your muscles grew bigger and stronger. The original weight became easier to lift, and soon you could hoist heavier loads. A similar process occurs as you make a change in your behavior. The first steps feel awkward and uncertain, but they become fluid and stronger with time and practice.

FAQ: *Why Are Some People Afraid to Change?*

Perhaps the greatest misconception about—and barrier to—personal change is the notion that you have to change who you *are*. You don't. The problem never is and never will be who you are. The problem—and what you need to change—is what you *do*.

The idea of who you are resides at the center of your sense of reality. It is part of the glue that holds your reality together. You believe that if you know anything, you know yourself. And you feel that you know what is possible for you.

What you actually know is what you have habitually believed and how you have consistently behaved. You have what police call an *m.o.,* or *modus operandi,* a way of doing things and a way of thinking about things that seldom varies in significant ways unless you consciously decide otherwise. You tie your shoes the same way, part your hair on the same side, lead with the same foot as you step into the shower, and rerun the same habitual thoughts and feelings through your brain.

When asked to attempt something different or new, you may think you can't do it on the basis of your past history. You mistake what you are unaccustomed to for something you cannot do. If you've never habitually been punctual, you can't see yourself suddenly being regularly on time. If you've always been disorganized, you can't imagine a clutter-free workspace. If you've gorged on junk food for years, you don't think a salad could ever satisfy you. If you fly off the handle at every slight, your temper seems untamable.

But life consists of doing things you never did before and of beginning to do them before you are sure you can. No rehearsal completely prepares you for the first day at a new school, a championship game, a driving test, or an admissions interview. Preparation helps, but there is a moment—often not entirely at your discretion—when you must deliver without the comforting sense of familiarity of having done so before. The experience can be scary, but it is the key to growing and moving forward with your life.

Remember that you, with all your talents and quirks, your passions and preferences, are more than the sum of your habits. You can change habits and not only retain the sense of who you are, but moreover experience the exhilaration of being the best and most complete version of you.

The Stages of Change

Psychologists have developed many theories about why we do the things we do. Some theories emphasize the role of the unconscious; others focus on the dynamics of our relationships or our thoughts and habits. Psychologist James Prochaska and his colleagues, by tracking what they considered universal stages in the successful recovery of drug addicts and alcoholics, developed a way of thinking about change that cuts across psychological theories. Their "transtheoretical" model focuses on universal aspects of an individual's decision-making process rather than on social or biological influences on behavior.

Instead of conceptualizing change as an exertion of effort or will, Prochaska identified various stages that people move through as they progress from being clueless, to conscious, to committed to making a change. This process begins slowly before you make a deliberate decision to change. Rather than marching in linear fashion from one stage to the next, most people spiral through the following stages.

Precontemplation

You are at this stage if you, as yet, have no intention of making a change. Even though you sense that something is not quite right or not quite the way you want it to be, you haven't identified exactly what's wrong, let alone thought about looking for solutions. You are vaguely uncomfortable, but this is where your grasp of what is going on ends. If you feel healthy and are busy with your classes and activities, for instance, you may never think about exercise. Then you notice that it's harder to zip your jeans or that you get winded walking up stairs. Still, you don't quite register the need to do anything about it.

During precontemplation, change remains hypothetical, distant, and vague and seems unlikely. Yet you may speak of something bugging you and wish that things were somehow different. If you ignore or override this discomfort or find sufficient distractions, precontemplation can last indefinitely and you won't change.

Contemplation

In this stage, you begin to get it. You acknowledge that something is amiss and begin to consider what it is and whether you can do anything about it. You still prefer not to have to change, but you start to realize that you can't avoid reality. Maybe none of your jeans fit anymore or you feel sluggish and listless. As you begin to weigh the trade-offs of standing pat versus acting, you may alternate between wanting to take action and resisting it. You may question your ability to change and feel moody and irritable.

The way you talk to yourself expresses your feeling that change is necessary but demonstrates your lack of commitment to taking action. Here are some examples of how the contemplation stage sounds:

- "I've got to do something about this."
- "I can't go on this way."
- "I hate it that I keep...."
- "I should...."
- "Maybe I can ride this out without having to change."
- "Maybe I'll do it someday—not tomorrow, but someday."

Each of these statements reveals the ambivalence and indecisiveness characteristic of the contemplation period. ("Your Line in the Sand," an exercise on page 35, can help you move beyond contemplation.)

Preparation

At some point you stop waffling, make a clear decision, and feel a burst of energy. This decision heralds the preparation stage. You gather information, make phone calls, do research online, and look into exercise classes at the gym. You begin to think and act with change specifically in mind, even if you hold something back.

Part of preparation is becoming internally accustomed to the idea of change and the impact it will make on you. This takes the form of mental rehearsal as you imagine what life will be like when you change. Trying things on for size in your mind helps you ready yourself to deal with higher expectations and new demands. In this phase you face your fears openly.

If you eavesdrop on what you're saying to yourself, you would hear statements such as "I am going to do this," and you would set a date, such as "I will begin on New Year's Day." Yet you may not share your plans with others. Despite all the internal progress you've made, you aren't necessarily ready to go completely public.

Action

This is the stage of actively modifying your behavior according to your plan. Your resolve is strong, and you know you're on your way to a better you. You no longer keep your plan under wraps—not that you could. Change produces signs that are visible to others. You may be getting up 15 minutes earlier to make time for a healthy breakfast or to walk to class rather than taking the shuttle.

In the action stage, things you mulled over and incubated for years unfold quickly. The more attention you devote to nurturing and solidifying your new habits, the faster they fall into place. In a relatively short time, you acquire a sense of comfort and ease with the change in your life.

Maintenance

Maintenance is about locking in and consolidating gains. This stabilizing stage, which follows the flurry of specific steps taken in the action stage, is necessary to retain what you've worked for and to make change permanent. Although at first it may sound as dull as changing oil and rotating tires, maintenance is an active, vital phase of the change process that provides the final ingredient needed for permanently reshaping your life. In this stage, you strengthen, enhance, and extend the changes you've initiated. You bring the rest of what you do into line with the change to support it. By securing the progress you've made, even if you hit a plateau or slip backward, you can regain your footing and keep moving forward.

FAQ: *Do I Need Willpower to Change?*

No. Willpower sounds like something you either have or don't have. Drop this idea. It is not useful. It is true that you need to make a resolute decision and take the steps necessary. But lack of willpower is not the culprit when people don't change; lack of knowledge is. Failure to change occurs when you choose the wrong tools or underestimate the length of time required for results to show. If you don't understand how change works, you may give up on the very brink of success. If so, don't blame willpower, which is nothing more than a set of habits that anyone can learn. You don't need to try harder; you need to be smarter about what change requires.

Although you must be motivated to change, this doesn't mean gritting your teeth with determination to change at all costs. Doing so actually distracts you from the work of personal change. Instead, focus on the pleasure you are moving toward and even on the pleasure of the process. When you devote yourself fully to something you want—something truly worth doing—you reap the extraordinary satisfaction and pleasure of directing your own life and becoming more accomplished.

The Joys of Mastery

If you ever spent time in another country or if your family immigrated to the United States, you know what it's like to find yourself immersed in a foreign world. Something as simple as taking a bus turns into a complex, mystifying challenge. You can't understand what people around you are saying. Even if you studied the native language in school, you may not be able to make yourself understood. You get so lost on streets with names you can't pronounce that you end up walking in circles.

But if you stay at it long enough and pay enough attention, you begin to get your bearings. You figure out where to buy bus tokens. You communicate with more than hand gestures. You memorize the route home and dare to ask directions if you need help. Each tiny triumph fills you with such glee that you silently applaud yourself. Such are the joys of rising to a challenge, daring to stretch yourself, and mastering something new and different.

Regardless of how old you are, whether you're at a small private school or a huge state university, whatever your ethnic background or economic status, college can seem a foreign universe. You may be living with strangers, eating unfamiliar foods, and struggling to figure out where you need to be when. You may have been a straight-A student, a varsity athlete, or editor of the high school newspaper, but that's no longer anything special—so were many of your new classmates. Everything that defined you in the past is gone. None of the old rules and routines apply. You have no choice but to change. This also means you have many new opportunities to earn and savor the joys of mastery.

We've leveled with you about the challenges of personal change. We've warned you to brace yourself for some turbulence because you will feel unsteady and uncertain and may be tempted to fall back on old behaviors. We've cautioned that you'll wonder if your efforts will pay off.

Here is another truth: They will.

As you will discover, when you make just one small, well-selected change, you open the door to more change. Change builds on itself. As you acquire essential basic skills in managing your life—the master skills and practices we describe in the next chapter—you gain a greater sense of mastery and become more capable of changing. Through this process you develop a new awareness of your inner responsibility for your life, your health, your body, your relationships, your achievements, and your future. Although you remain your true self, you also become something more: a successful personal change agent—in other words, a successful director of your life story.

In the process, you will find plenty of things to learn—and to like. Be a sponge. Soak up knowledge. You are happiest when you are learning because humans are wired this way. You raise the ante on adventure the moment you begin to direct change. You feel most alive when you stretch yourself. Although you have a destination, you will pass through unexplored territory on the way, and you can count on the unexpected. If you fear you cannot progress beyond some level, look again. You can do it. You are becoming a master.

Your Mega-Horsepower Change Machine

When you direct personal change, you take advantage of the most powerful resource on the planet: the human mind. Your mind is more than your brain. Whereas the brain is an amazing information-processing machine, the mind is the sense of consciousness and of choice that arises out of it. And change changes your mind, not just your brain. As you read the information and practice the exercises in this book and the *IPC Labs,* the way you think about yourself will change, the way you feel about yourself will change, and your behaviors will change.

Remember: You have the capacity and the option to choose. But you have to be aware of opportunities for change in order to act on them. Otherwise, choice points come and go and you do not take advantage of them. By default you respond in the ways you always have and you stay largely the same.

An Invitation to Personal Change will show you how to become aware of your choices. One of its lessons is how to peer into and monitor your mind. You will become conscious of the words, phrases, and messages you use to talk to yourself. You will step back from yourself and "see," perhaps for the first time, the ways in which you make choices that don't always serve you well and how the language you use either unlocks possibilities or puts up barriers. You will become aware of your thoughts at the moment you are thinking them. If necessary, you will learn to work with them, rearrange them, or replace them with more effective, less limiting thoughts. This is what it means to direct change.

As you take control of your thoughts and behavior, you will no longer drift mindlessly through the day. You will take more positive actions and engage in fewer activities you later regret. You will consciously and unconsciously alter your brain and your mind. You will think differently about your choices. And by changing your choices, you will direct change in your life.

real change: clueless on campus

After her first month in college, Alejandra feels overwhelmed—and then some. She is thousands of miles from home, family, friends, and familiar faces and foods. Her dormmates range from different to downright difficult. Her professors expect her to read and learn more in a week than she did in an entire month of high school. Always a strong B+ student, she got a D+ on her first college paper.

Because of her tight budget, Alejandra is living on 99-cent burritos and noodles that she heats in the microwave and eats straight from the Styrofoam cup. Watching frat guys play beer pong isn't her idea of a fun evening, but she doesn't want to stay alone in her room on a Saturday night. Afterward she regrets wasting so much time.

Alejandra knows she doesn't have her footing yet. She feels disoriented, but she doesn't know what to do about it. The idea of pulling things together seems beyond reach. She is scrambling to do everything the best she can. What could she, would she, should she change? Just go home? No way. She couldn't. She knows she has to get her bearings, and she needs to change something or maybe many things. The question is what and how to find the time.

You can follow Alejandra's story from her current stage of precontemplation to directing change in her life in Chapter 4.

real change: second time around

Nate, 36, is twice as old as the youngest student in his class—and, he hopes, twice as wise. His first time at college, he didn't want to waste what he saw as his prime partying years in a study cubicle. He'd sailed through high school without working up much of an intellectual sweat. Expecting to ace his first-year classes, he was shocked to find himself barely passing most of them.

By sophomore year Nate was on academic probation. When he found a good-paying job in construction the next summer, he decided to stick with it rather than return to campus. "Not everybody's cut out for college," he told his friends and family. "I can make a good living without a degree."

Nate's no longer sure of that. Whenever the housing market slumped or a big retail development ran out of funds, he lost his job. By scrambling from crew to crew, he was usually able to pick up work. With two small kids, job security became more important than ever. But money wasn't the only drawback. As Nate got older, back and shoulder problems began to plague him. He couldn't imagine spending the rest of his life pounding nails.

Nate started saving money and taking courses at night school. He's back at school part time, but he's worried about the challenge. Drinking and partying have lost all appeal, but Nate wonders if he's too old to learn new material. Is his brain up to it? At times Nate feels so overwhelmed that he thinks he's running in circles, getting and going nowhere.

To find out how Nate finds his focus, see the continuation of this Real Change in Chapter 8.

Personal Change 101

Think of the last time you changed your look. Maybe you tried a new haircut or hair color or decided to make a fashion statement for a special occasion. Even these superficial changes didn't happen in the blink of an eye. All required a decision, a plan, and action. You probably spent quite a bit of time considering how you might look with your hair shorter or lighter. Before settling on a new outfit, you may have trekked through half a dozen stores.

When you took the plunge, the results may or may not have lived up to your expectations. But at the least you learned from your experiment—if only to steer clear of magenta highlights or to never get another buzz cut. Most importantly, you looked at yourself in a different way.

Opening your eyes and your mind to new, sometimes surprising possibilities is part of change's thrill—and terror. When restlessness drives you to the brink of change, you feel ready to break out of your rut. At the same time, all you know is how you have done things so far. Like blinders, your past experiences limit your vision. You look at life through the lens of your preexisting ideas and biases. To change you have to set aside these preconceptions and expand your sense of your possibilities.

You also have to be ready to roll up your sleeves and do some work. If change were as simple as snapping your fingers, you would have already transformed yourself. As we've said, change—real, lasting change—requires commitment and effort. Taking personal responsibility is essential. If you decide that you don't want or need to behave responsibly, you will not change. If you blame other people or circumstances for what's wrong in your life, you will remain stuck where you are.

Change is a learning process. You have been learning and changing all your life, so this is not new, complicated, or overwhelming. But you must take some time to get ready to change. If do not prepare well, if you are not open and flexible, and if you do not pay close attention, you undermine your attempts to change. Like a carpenter who doesn't take time to measure properly, your best efforts won't produce the results you had hoped for. This chapter, which introduces the underlying components of successful change, prepares you to make change happen more efficiently and effectively.

To prepare for learning and understanding more about change, answer the self-survey in the following box. After completing it, continue with the text to find out how the scale was developed and what it means.

Are You Internal or External?

Depending on which statement you agree with, check either a or b for each of the following.

1. (a) Many of the unhappy things in people's lives are partly due to bad luck. ____
   (b) People's misfortunes result from the mistakes they make. ____
2. (a) One of the major reasons why we have wars is because people don't take enough interest in politics. ____
   (b) There will always be wars, no matter how hard people try to prevent them. ____
3. (a) In the long run, people get the respect they deserve in this world. ____
   (b) Unfortunately, an individual's worth often passes unrecognized no matter how hard he tries. ____
4. (a) The idea that teachers are unfair to students is nonsense. ____
   (b) Most students don't realize the extent to which their grades are influenced by accidental happenings. ____
5. (a) Without the right breaks, one cannot be an effective leader. ____
   (b) Capable people who fail to become leaders have not taken advantage of their opportunities. ____
6. (a) No matter how hard you try, some people just don't like you. ____
   (b) People who can't get others to like them don't understand how to get along with others. ____
7. (a) I have often found that what is going to happen will happen. ____
   (b) Trusting to fate has never turned out as well for me as making a decision to take a definite course of action. ____
8. (a) In the case of the well-prepared student, there is rarely, if ever, such a thing as an unfair test. ____
   (b) Many times exam questions tend to be so unrelated to course work that studying is really useless. ____
9. (a) Becoming a success is a matter of hard work; luck has little or nothing to do with it. ____
   (b) Getting a good job depends mainly on being in the right place at the right time. ____
10. (a) The average citizen can have influence in government decisions. ____
    (b) This world is run by the few people in power, and there is not much the little guy can do about it. ____
11. (a) When I make plans, I am almost certain that I can make them work. ____
    (b) It is not always wise to plan too far ahead because many things turn out to be a matter of luck anyway. ____
12. (a) In my case, getting what I want has little or nothing to do with luck. ____
    (b) Many times we might just as well decide what to do by flipping a coin. ____
13. (a) What happens to me is my own doing. ____
    (b) Sometimes I feel that I don't have enough control over the direction my life is taking. ____

Scoring: Give yourself one point for each of the following answers:
1a, 2b, 3b, 4b, 5a, 6a, 7a, 8b, 9b, 10b, 11b, 12b, 13 b

You do not get any points for other choices.

Add up the totals. Scores can range from 0 to 13. A high score indicates an external locus of control, the belief that forces outside yourself control your destiny. A low score indicates an internal locus of control, a belief in your ability to take charge of your life.

Source: Based on Rotter, J.B. "Generalized Expectancies for Internal versus External Control of Reinforcement," *Psychological Monographs*, vol. 80, whole no. 609 (1966).

Taking Control

Decades ago in a university laboratory, volunteers played a game. They sat in front of a panel containing three buttons. Below the buttons was a round hole from which marbles rolled into a small trough. Their goal was to try to win as many marbles as possible by pressing the buttons on the panel.

Some "contestants" were told this was a game of chance and it made no difference which buttons they pressed. Others were told that this was a game of skill and that their strategic pushing of the buttons would determine the outcome. The volunteers didn't know that, no matter which buttons they pressed in which order, they all received marbles in the same fixed, predetermined sequence. At some point the marbles stopped coming. What happened then?

The volunteers who thought they were playing a game of chance played for a while then quit. What was the point of continuing? Those told the game depended on their skill not only kept playing but also repeatedly changed tactics and tried complicated strategies, as if trying to remember which actions had produced marbles before.

Psychologist Julian Rotter, who devised this now-classic experiment, wondered whether the results might tell us something about people's conceptions about life. Some people, he theorized, go about life as if they received "skill" instructions for it, while others feel nothing they do will make any difference. His hunch was that if people viewed outcomes as directly related to their efforts, they would persist longer, try harder, and apply their intelligence to solving a problem—just like the participants in his game of marbles.

Rotter's observations led to more than 30 years of research into locus of control, the sense of what determines what happens in life. "Internals" assume they are personally responsible for what happens to them; "externals" view their lives as governed by luck or fate. Internals who get an A on a test credit their hard work and understanding of the material, while Externals assume the teacher was an easy grader or used a curve. Internals in general act more independently, enjoy better health, and are more optimistic about their future. Externals find it harder to cope with stress and feel increasingly helpless over time.

In our research, we've found that an internal locus of control also is related to higher self-esteem. Self-esteem has to do not just with feeling good about yourself but also with achieving results. You cannot and do not achieve results if you do not act and if you are not willing to change. On the other hand, you will not exert effort unless you have a reasonable expectation of being able to succeed. An internal locus of control sets up a positive spiral that builds on itself.

To the extent that you see yourself as in control or under control of others, you obtain the results you expect. This is the impact of expectations and projections. We constantly receive what we expect from others and from life, largely because our actions evoke from others the responses we anticipate. Whether we realize it or not, we do not merely hold expectations: We also communicate them. Our expectations sit in the driver's seat. But if we consciously choose our expectations? Then we direct our lives.

Do you see yourself—at least to some significant degree—as the master of your fate, asserting control over your destiny? Or does your life seem so chaotic that you just hang on and hope for the best? Either way, your expectations have two effects: They filter what you notice or ignore in your daily experiences, and they announce to the world what you anticipate. Both affect how others respond to you. Since people assume that you know more than they do about who you are and what you can do, they take their cues from you. If you act as if control is not yours, someone will rush to fill the vacuum.

If you turned out to be external on the self-assessment quiz on page 15, don't accept your current score as a given for life. If you want to shift your perspective, you can. People are not internal or external in every situation. At home you may go along with your parents' or roommates' preferences and let them call the shots. In class you might feel confident and participate without hesitation.

Take inventory of the situations in which you feel most and least in control. Are you bold on the basketball court but hesitant on a date? Do you feel confident that you can resolve a dispute with your friends but throw up your hands when a landlord refuses to refund your security deposit? Look for ways to exert more influence in situations in which you once yielded to external influences. See what a difference you can make.

Believing You Can

Feeling in control goes hand in hand with believing in your ability to change. In his groundbreaking research, psychologist Albert Bandura of Stanford University found that the individuals most likely to reach a goal are those who believe that they can. Your judgment of your self-efficacy helps determine whether you undertake particular goal-directed activities. Your sense of self-efficacy also determines the amount of effort you put into these attempts and the length of time you persist in striving. Sound like internal locus of control? The results are similar.

A strong sense of self-efficacy provides another bonus: a calming effect in situations that involve threat or hazards. Confronted with danger, individuals with little faith in their abilities become anxious and panic. Catastrophic thoughts flood their brains. By comparison, a sense of self-efficacy reduces anxiety and stimulates thinking about effective action.

The stronger your faith in your ability to succeed, the less fear you will feel and the more energy and persistence you will put into making a change. The opposite is also true, especially for health behaviors. In one study of people who began an exercise program, those with a lower sense of self-efficacy were more likely to drop out. They didn't believe that they could or would reach their goals, so they gave up before they had a chance to succeed.

What if you feel that your sense of self-efficacy is low? For now, take it as truth that it *will* change in the same way that locus of control changes. With the new information we provide to guide you, you will experience new achievements that will help you reach new conclusions about your possibilities.

FAQ: *What Causes Resistance to Change?*

Whether we view change as positive or not, necessary or not, even welcome or not, we often initially resist. Much of this resistance stems from preconceptions. Facing new information is like coming out of the darkness you were accustomed to and walking into intense light. Reflexively, you squint or close your eyes and turn toward the comfort of darkness. You have to give your brain time to adjust, just as your pupils need time to respond to bright light.

Resistance is especially strong when change threatens to alter what you believe about yourself based on past experiences. The more you believe change is impossible, the more you will make it so. The more you know about what is possible and essential for change, the less resistance you will create. Often people have a distorted sense of how much effort will be involved in giving up what they are sure of in order to do something new and different. They anticipate more difficulty than they experience once they push past resistance and get going with the actual steps and tasks associated with change.

If you encounter resistance, recognize it as an indicator of strength—exactly the kind of strength you need to sustain change. Remember: If it were possible for you to change easily, you would just as easily lose valuable skills you worked hard to perfect. What would you do if you suddenly lost your ability to skateboard, read music, or simply fry an egg? You would scurry to a neurologist's office to find out what was wrong with your brain.

Your brain and your body naturally hang on to habits they've learned. This is good. The more tenaciously you stay locked into habits, the more robust the health of your overall nervous system. Don't fight this. It is how you are constructed. Resistance is negative only if you use it as an excuse to abandon your effort. Instead, accept it for what it is: a temporary phase in the process of personal change.

Under the Influence: Social Norms and You

Freshmen arriving on the campus of a large California university puzzled over the phrase on the T-shirts worn by sophomore "greeters" at their dormitories: 0 to 3. Was it the score of last year's homecoming game? An inside joke? A local band? The answer was none of the above. "0 to 3" is the number of drinks that surveys showed the average student consumes at a party.

So why was the message put on the T-shirts? The T-shirts campaign was a simple way of communicating clear information about actual statistics on college drinking. The reason? In recent years colleges have found that publicizing research data on behaviors such as drinking, smoking, and drug use helps students develop a more accurate sense of campus social norms—the behaviors that any group expects, accepts, supports, or considers normal and important.

When the media speak of a youth culture or business consultants talk about corporate cultures, they are describing how groups of people, out of a sense of belonging or wanting to belong, function according to distinctive rules. As social animals, we measure ourselves and our behaviors according to various yardsticks provided by reference groups—the groups we consider ourselves to be part of. Surgeons measure their success against other surgeons, bricklayers against other bricklayers.

Leaving your family and finding a new social network at college or at your first job are crucial parts of your development. In any new situation, conforming, to some degree, to general expectations can serve as a shortcut to fitting in and gaining acceptance or feeling a sense of belonging.

But research demonstrates that perceptions about social norms are often skewed. This may be especially true on college campuses, where undergraduates often misjudge what their peers are—and aren't—doing. Only anonymous responses to a scientifically designed questionnaire can reveal what students do—the *actual* social norms—compared to what they may say they do in order to gain social approval.

For instance, in the American College Health Association's National College Health Assessment, which has surveyed hundreds of thousands undergraduates at schools across the country, about two-thirds said they had never smoked cigarettes—yet they guessed that only 10 percent of college students had done the same. Only 0.4 percent of students surveyed report drinking alcohol every day, but undergraduates think 37 percent do so.

Students who arrive on a campus with a reputation as a party school may immediately assume that their peers are all drinking heavily, using drugs, or engaging in risky sexual behaviors. To fit in, they may say they do the same, even if they don't, thereby helping perpetuate the myth.

Would you do something solely because "everyone" seems to be doing it? We hope not. Although it would be great if all students developed independent values and were unafraid to live by them, it takes longer for some than for others to do so. That's why knowing true social norms matters.

FAQ: *When Is the Best Time to Make a Change?*

Now. Trust us on this. If you wait for change to happen spontaneously or for circumstances to change, you will keep waiting. Hoping fortune will come and smile upon you is not a method for change. Fortune has already smiled and given you the present moment.

Postponing change is not simply postponing; it is failure to act. Any apparent advantage usually turns out to be imaginary. If you wait until you have more money or more time, or until you're comfortable with what the future holds, you may end up waiting forever. If you wait to be in the right mood to change, you inevitably will wait longer than necessary. To change, you need something other than time, money, or a certain mood. You need master skills, the skills we describe later in this chapter.

On the other hand, rather than waiting for the perfect time to come, you may fear that your ideal moment has passed. Think again. There is no one single moment, no one single choice, that defines a life. Believing that you missed your chance, believing that the time is not right or ripe for change, is a way to justify not changing. All of us have passed on important opportunities. If you keep looking back, you get yourself trapped in regret and ignore the opportunities that exist now. You cannot relive or undo the past, but you have this moment in time. You decide what you want to do with it.

What if you're too busy right now? Who isn't? No one has the time to change. You must steal it. Start small if you must, but start. Do not fall into the "if I can't exercise for an hour, I won't exercise at all" trap. If something is worth doing, it is worth doing for whatever amount of time you can give it. And it is worth starting now.

Turning Fear into an Ally

Ask people why they don't make a personal change, and the answer nearly always boils down to the same thing: fear. They hunker down and hold fast to their current position, even if it is not an ideal or a healthy one. Fear immobilizes them and makes them rein in what they might otherwise try. They are afraid of the unknown, afraid of failing, afraid of embarrassing themselves, afraid of discovering they do not have what it takes, or afraid that if they change, people will expect more of them. What they're really saying is that if not for their fear, they would make significant changes. The implication is that fear is what stops them.

Blaming fear also suggests that people who boldly make changes and take on daring challenges must do so because they don't experience fear. This simply isn't true. Those who push the envelope and venture beyond their comfort zones are not necessarily fearless. They take fear seriously for what it is—a signal to use caution. If you feel fear, begin to investigate its source.

If you fear something, it is because you perceive danger. Good. It's far better to perceive danger than to ignore it. People unable to perceive danger wind up getting hurt through ignorance or recklessness. On the other hand, never allow fear or the existence of danger alone to stop you in your tracks. Instead of running for cover, realize that where there is danger, you must be appropriately cautious. Danger requires (1) you think beyond "Wouldn't it be a rush to....?" before deciding to proceed and (2) you take reasonable precautions before acting. Driving a car or striking a match carries a risk of danger, but you don't avoid either. Instead, you heighten your attention so that you do them safely.

If you work with fear correctly, it will become your ally. Let fear prompt you to take appropriate precautions. Don't leap before looking, but don't retreat before finding out what to expect. Get information. Doing so is the only way to determine whether a danger is real and what specific threat it presents. Don't cringe. Giving in to fear leads to mindlessly freezing in your tracks. If you let that happen, your life will be safe and predictable—but barren. A certain level of fear can inform and motivate you and can alert you to authentic hazards. Then you can evaluate and decide what level of daring makes sense.

The downside of fear is that, if not handled appropriately, it has a way of making your worst nightmare come true. When you're afraid of something, you try to avoid it—and whenever you do so, you are more likely to experience what you fear most. Picture yourself standing on the free throw line to shoot two foul shots. Your team is one point behind with one second left on the clock. If you shoot hoping not to blow the shot, you are more likely to miss than if you shoot saying to yourself, "These guys are toast!" The reason? When you worry about failure rather than going on the offensive, your fear creates muscular tension that disrupts the fluidity of your shot.

The same thing happens whenever you have to do something you dread, such as speaking in public. If you have to make a presentation in class, focusing on not making a fool of yourself is the kiss of death. Even if you do a great deal of research and feel passionately about the subject, you are far less likely to give a good talk if you are trying to avoid giving a bad one. Concentrate instead on what you want to say and what you want people to understand. Tell yourself that you have something wonderful to share with everyone in your audience and that it is your luck and theirs that you have this time together.

FAQ: *What If I'm Too Lazy or Stubborn to Change?*

Maybe you say you're just lazy. All of us are—or can be. Laziness exists inside us, alongside traits such as ambition and energy. If you give laziness sway, it will take over your life. But you are more than any single trait, positive or negative. Remember, as director of the film, you run the show. Making a personal change is a decision. You can tell your cast of traits what you want and when you want them to make an appearance. Let laziness reign during spring break, but limit it to a walk-on cameo in your daily life.

Your less desirable characteristics will get in the way of change only if you let them. Say that you have a stubborn streak. Stubbornness in one situation translates into tenacity in another. Get stubborn about reaching a new goal or directing the changes you want in some habit. In other words, put your stubbornness to work on behalf of a new cause. Turn your attributes around in this manner, and you will see more clearly the possibilities that exist within your so-called liabilities.

There are advantages and disadvantages in all your characteristics. Finding the positive within your negative habits is worth doing. It allows you to work with everything you bring to the dance. Remember what we said earlier: You do not need to change who you are. This is one of the areas in which this is true. You will back away from change quickly if you criticize yourself for being who you are. If you are inclined to be self-critical, stop going there. Resist attacking yourself with dire interpretations of the mistakes you feel you have made. That was then. This is now. Move on.

The Master Skills and Practices of Personal Change

Master skills and practices are habits you can apply to every activity or task—academic, athletic, professional, or personal. You have a set of discrete skills and habits related to, say, blow-drying your hair. You take out the dryer, turn it on high (never low or medium), and use a brush so that your hair dries full and straight. Your actions are habitual and do not require great thought or attention. Blow-drying your hair is not in itself a master skill. But master skills and practices govern the care and attention with which you approach any other activity, whether polishing your shoes or researching a paper. They affect the outcome—as you know if you ever lived through a bad hair day after a rushed or botched blow-dry.

You began acquiring master skills long ago—at the piano bench, in the dance studio, on the soccer field or playground. Although you focused on the task at hand, you were always learning more. Master skills such as patience, whether acquired by playing scales or the discipline of shot selection, are invaluable because you can apply them again and again to new situations. They increase your capacity for change and lay the foundation for developing all kinds of new, more complex habits and skills.

Bypass lessons in the master skills, and you pay a price. You probably know kids who tried to dodge the anxiety and awkwardness of adolescent relationships by taking drugs. Their "solution" only created more problems. With their social and academic development arrested, some became trapped in dead-ends they may never escape.

The mastery of master skills is a win–win proposition. As you direct a personal change, you build and strengthen your master skills. And as your master skills grow, they make the process of personal change more efficient. Here are some key skills that the exercises in Part II and the *Labs for An Invitation to Personal Change* will help you develop.

Order

We're not your mom, and we're not telling you to clean up your room. But we will tell you a secret: Living without order means being out of control. Order is the path to true efficiency. Rushing and improvising bring disorder, and disorder makes slaves of us. Whatever disorder you leave behind today will steal part of tomorrow from you. Put aside the notion that carrying a day planner or keeping a to-do list is something only a parent, teacher, or incorrigible nerd would do. If you want to take control of your time (and therefore your future), the first thing you have to do is put your life in order. (The exercises in Chapter 5 are a good place to start.)

Focusing Attention

All of us—not just those who may have been told they have attention deficit disorder—have problems paying attention. This is no accident. The capacity to be distracted may have saved our species. If our prehistoric ancestors weren't distracted by a charging wooly mastodon as they gathered berries or tended a fire, we wouldn't be here today.

In today's mastodon-free world, you know how to focus attention on things that are exciting or enticing. Your mind doesn't wander when you're gaming with your friends or, for that matter, when you're kissing (well, maybe when you're kissing). If your attention lapses when you're studying Spanish verb conjugations or memorizing chemistry formulas, however, you may blame boredom. Actually, it's the other way around. Boredom is often a sign that you have withdrawn your attention. This can be dangerous—particularly if you're behind the wheel and suddenly realize you've driven for miles without noticing your surroundings.

When you withdraw attention from other activities, you miss opportunities for learning and for exercising choice. As we have already said, not noticing that you have a choice effectively takes away your chance to choose. The meditation traditions of both the East and the West were developed to harness attention in order to create more opportunities for personal mastery. Solving a difficult equation or memorizing the lines of a play also provides opportunities for concentrating attention. Without attention, you may not, for example, notice a strategy you could employ to solve a personal problem or the inconvenience your actions may be causing someone else.

Contemporary brain research demonstrates that if you learn something new you actually change the structure of the brain. But here is the kicker: If you learn something so well that you go on autopilot while doing it, brain growth for that activity stops. So when you are not paying attention, you are not using your highest brain functions, not developing your highest capacities, and not cashing in on the benefit of your evolutionary heritage. (Several of the exercises in the *IPC Labs* can help enhance your attention.)

For a variety of reasons, from cultural to religious, you may feel that meditation is not for you. However, if you consider meditation as focusing and infuse everything, even actions you once considered monotonous, with exaggerated attention you not only grow your brain capacity but also transform your experience and often make the actions themselves more meaningful. (For more on meditation, see the "Rx: Relax" lab in the *IPC Labs*.)

Develop the habit of drenching with attention any experience you consider boring. The next time you're sitting through a dull lecture, for instance, pay more attention rather than less. Focus on exactly why the professor's talk is so tedious. Think of ways you could make every aspect of the presentation more interesting—or even more boring. Doing this forces you to pay more attention. As a result, you use the opportunity presented by the boring lecture to strengthen a master skill: your capacity to direct and focus your attention. You also redeem time that would have been wasted, and you feel fresher and sharper.

Persistence

Persistence means continuing to work and to keep moving forward, no matter what. A lack of persistence leads to the failure of many worthwhile ventures that, if only given more time, would eventually have borne fruit. You do not go from photography student to Pulitzer Prize winner in a year. You do not go from sketching a skirt to launching your own clothing line in 18 months. You need to persist long enough to give new and creative ideas sufficient time to take root.

You would not be reading this if not for your proven persistence. How many times did you stumble over words before you could pronounce and understand them? Before that, how many times did you fall on your bottom before you could toddle across a room? Hundreds. It was no big deal. You just kept falling and failing until you got the hang of upright locomotion.

Problems with persistence crop up later in life, after your ego becomes attached to not making mistakes or not wanting to humiliate yourself by failing yet again. The more skills you accumulate and the more you become accustomed to success, the more allergic you can become to feeling inadequate or unskilled—sensations that come with the territory of change.

Because change can feel shaky in its early stages, you need persistence to pull you through what ski instructors call "the valley of doom." Novice skiers often observe that after taking a lesson devoted to learning a new technique they ski worse for a while. The reason is they are leaving behind the familiar groove of automatic habits and having to "think."

Change produces the same effect. If you don't recognize this, you may abandon a change campaign because your initial efforts seem to be setting you back rather than moving you forward. But if you do not persist, you will remain stuck where you are. This is why the master skill of persistence is so essential.

Take a pointer from professional golfer Tiger Woods. On two separate occasions during his professional career after winning numerous championships, Woods deliberately decided to change his swing. This was radical—and controversial. Why would a winner tamper with success? Woods was convinced that the changes would ultimately raise his game and contribute to the longevity of his career. So he took a risk and paid a price. Both times, his game fell off for nearly two years. But on both occasions, after the dip in performance he played better than ever. To take such a risk he had to have a strong sense of self-efficacy. But to accomplish his goals he had to persist in the face of negative results.

Consistency

Although all-nighters are one approach to finals, every scientific study of learning has demonstrated that regular, consistent, spaced intervals of practice produce the greatest gains. Inconsistent effort usually yields haphazard results. At times you may need a big burst of effort—or more than one—to push a particular project to completion. But individuals who consistently achieve usually develop a methodical set of routines that enable them to make and keep making a focused effort over time.

The words *kung fu* translate into "consistent practice over time." A tennis serve or a brush stroke in calligraphy can be *kung fu* because it is the product of repeated practice. Even the most creative artists and writers—and certainly dancers and athletes—know that they have to put in regular effort to stay at the top of what they do. To learn new skills, to direct and make change, requires the same. It is as simple as that. If you want to produce quality changes with the least amount of total effort, you must master the skill of consistency.

Repetition

When you learned to direct a soccer ball with a header, successfully make a backward somersault off the high dive, or flirt discreetly, you practiced repetitively even if you did not think of it that way at the time. Whether you took classical dance lessons or became a water polo goalie, you likewise engaged in intense repetitive practice. If you practiced because you took personal pleasure from making progress, you undoubtedly made more progress faster.

Successful repetition is not a matter of forcing yourself to repeat an action but a matter of tuning into the process. Much impatience stems from focusing on end points and outcomes rather than the steps leading to them. When things are worth doing well, all parts are worth doing. You do not go to a concert to hear the encore. If you persist at anything, you increase your ability to persist, tolerate frustration and monotony, and continue to work despite setbacks.

Because learning new skills requires repetition, learn to love it. Although it is thrilling to grasp things quickly and do remarkable things effortlessly, skills that demand repetition yield a different kind of pleasure. Do not miss out on this enjoyment. If you duck out of language labs or hockey practices, you cheat yourself of opportunities to master repetition. By taking pleasure in these sessions, you will progress more rapidly. Try this out and see for yourself.

Developing patience through repetition is the master skill equivalent of physical reps in the weight room. Each delivers the cumulative power of small repeated actions. If you consider small acts trifles that are not worth the bother, you will remain unable to do large things. You must get in shape and build emotional endurance. Repetition builds internal muscle, which you can engage whenever you need to learn something new.

Finishing

Ask a novelist how it feels to write "The End" after months or years of slaving over a manuscript. The two little words yield the sweetest sense of satisfaction. You feel the same way when you paint the last backdrop for the spring play or complete your final lab for an advanced biochemistry class. As the Swiss philosopher Henri Frederic Amiel observed, "to finish is the mark of the master." Finishing also offers a great sense of mastery.

As long as anything remains to be done, nothing is really done. But did you ever notice that finishing something completely and well is in itself a skill? Some people finish everything but the last class for their major or the last test for their lifeguard certificate. Or they complete a degree or certificate and never pursue the career they prepared for. Why?

It is absolutely okay to change your mind about a career and to go in a different direction. But sometimes people stop short of completion because they fear that in some way whatever comes next will present some new challenge that they might not be able to meet. Or they fear that what they prepared for will be a disappointment. In response they avoid completion or endlessly procrastinate rather than find out.

An aspiring songwriter we know is always jotting down lyrics and opening chords but has never finished a single tune. She can play captivating bits of music but has never performed or recorded a complete song of her own. Her life, like too many others, is an unfinished symphony. Don't let your song go unsung, your music unheard. Master the skill of finishing what you begin.

Making Personal Change Inevitable

When you were little, change was a normal, everyday event. You amazed your parents with how quickly you changed—and you amazed yourself as you added remarkable feats like walking and talking to your repertoire. Children caught up in the magic of daily discoveries change without considering alternative ways of being. They try new things, fail where they will, pick themselves up, and try again.

At some point in life, for whatever reason, we start saying about some engrained habit, "It's just the way I am." That's not true. It's the way you *have done things until now*. Declaring that you can't change wastes time you could be using to make change inevitable. And change is inevitable—if you do the work.

The first step on the way to directing your life is to commit quietly but fully to a personal change and vow not to stop before reaching your goal. If you don't decide to change, your old habits win out. The moment you decide, you become formidable, like some hungry animal that will hunt relentlessly until it finds food. Things become clear. Life becomes simpler because when you decide, you simplify it. One priority rises to the top. Making an unequivocal choice for change unleashes a nearly unstoppable force, especially if you tune into the pleasure.

A decision to move from where you are requires a concrete plan. This may sound daunting, but you already have a grasp of how to go about it. If you ever plotted ahead of time how to tell your parents about your plan to backpack in Europe or how to get the attention of a cute classmate across the aisle, you have experience in setting out a plan. Making a plan concrete simply requires taking that kind of strategizing and elaborating on it.

No matter how complex a desired change may be, you can break it down into finite steps. Once you develop a step-by-step plan and consistently follow it, you can replace any habit, however tenacious. Nevertheless, for a while the new habit will have to compete with the old ingrained one. You will have to exert effort until you have locked in the new behavior.

Just as when you learned to swim, when you begin your first efforts to change, you may cling to the side of the pool or rely on artificial supports like water wings far longer than you need to. Both are ways of cheating yourself. At some point you have to give up what makes you feel secure in order to take the next step. You have to let go of the edge.

Change becomes inevitable if you persist even when you fear that you're in over your head and when your efforts seem to have no apparent effect other than hassling and irritating you. Change takes time, but usually only the early results are disconcerting.

Change tinkers with deeply entrenched habits and patterns of thinking that exist beyond your consciousness. You will have some temporary hell to pay for this disruption. But if you understand that new routines feel upsetting only until you become accustomed to them, you will persist in the face of challenges that otherwise might discourage you.

Any habit can be changed. Change is no mystery. You do the work, and you make the change. But you have to keep working until you do. Then you lock in the gains. This is what it means to finish: to go all the way.

real change: out of order

So far this week Noah has pulled one all-nighter, slept through his alarm two mornings in a row, missed the deadline for a class paper, and forgotten an appointment with his academic advisor. And it's only Wednesday!

"I don't know where the time goes," Noah complains. He tries to jot down what he's supposed to do, but then he loses the piece of paper. His roommate posts a calendar with his schedule and assignments above his desk. That is definitely not Noah's style. Some of his friends use their computers or PDAs to keep track of commitments, but Noah says he's never been much of a techie. He keeps planning to buy a day planner but never gets around to it. Besides, it probably would get buried under the books and papers heaped upon his desk—like the card he bought for his mom's birthday and forgot to send.

"If I just had more time I'd get organized," Noah tells himself. But when he looks at the clothes heaped on the closet floor, the Styrofoam containers from last weekend's takeout, and the books and papers piled on his desk, he shakes his head. Where would he even begin? And even if he could beat back the chaos, wouldn't the mess return like some movie swamp monster in a week or so?

You can find out whether Noah escapes the forces of disorder in Chapter 5.

real change: test terror

Malika didn't remember school being so hard. Of course, she'd spent most of the last four years changing diapers, soothing tantrums, and crooning lullabies to her twins. She doesn't regret taking time off to cherish their early years, but now she's ready to pick up her career dreams. Even though the girls are thriving at preschool, Malika worries about juggling their needs with a full academic load. But nothing scares her more than tests.

"Malika doesn't test well," she remembers her mother saying at parent–teacher conferences in high school. Fortunately, she usually did such an outstanding job on papers and projects that she could pull her grades up. But in college your entire grade can depend on a midterm and final exam. Malika has a recurring dream of opening a blue exam book and not being able to think of a single word to write.

Her first midterm turned into the disaster Malika feared. She couldn't sleep the night before. She didn't know if her hands were shaking because of anxiety or the four cups of coffee she chugged before the test. Her mind seemed to turn to glue. She passed—with a D. When she asked the teaching assistant what she could do to earn a better grade on the next test, he blew her off with a one-word answer: study! That only made Malika feel more inadequate and more anxious.

To find out how Malika deals with test stress, turn to the continuation of this Real Change in Chapter 9.

CHAPTER 3

The Story of You

The School of Life

FAQ: *Why Don't We Make Changes We Know Are Good for Us?*

Bad Risks, Good Risks: Knowing the Difference

FAQ: *Don't Most People Who Try to Change Give Up in a Few Months?*

Staying Healthy on Campus

FAQ: *What If I Blow It?*

Changing for Good

Real Change: Tomorrow Is Another Diet

Real Change: Off Track?

Classroom Activity: Your Line in the Sand

Journaling Assignment: Crossing the Line

Visualization: Crossing the Line

"Once upon a time…."

This is the way the tales we cherished as children begin. But there's another story that started years ago. It begins like this: "Once upon a time…. there was you."

As we've said, you are the director of your movie. You couldn't control where or when it began. For years your parents decided what you wore, what you ate, where you went to school, when you could watch television or play video games. But from an early age, you started doing the one thing no one else could: being yourself.

Maybe you were the girl who could outrun all the boys in her class. Maybe you were the boy who made everybody laugh. Maybe you were the quiet one, the musical one, the one who caught the most fish or knew all the state capitals. Or maybe you remember being the clumsy sibling who always spilled the milk, the chubby kid nobody wanted on the team, the tongue-tied geek who could never think of anything to say.

You cannot change the past. Unlike for a film, there are no dress rehearsals, second takes, or reshoots. Whatever plot turns your life has taken, you cannot literally go back and revise them. You may or may not want to; fortunately you do not have to. You can learn or do anything now that you did not learn or do in the past. You can change the direction of your story from this point forward.

College represents a new chapter. No one—parent, teacher, or resident adviser—is micromanaging your life. Most people in your classes never met you before. They don't know or care whether you lisped for years or won the junior high spelling bee. They see you as you are and judge you by what you do. College can be the dividing line between what was and what will be. Use this time to do what you—and only you—can: direct what happens next in the story of you.

The School of Life

The school of life doesn't charge tuition or grant degrees, but it does provide all elements that you *need* to learn and that you need *in order to* learn. What can you expect to learn in the school of life? Consider the experience of a man who sought help from a wise therapist we know.

His aim was to determine what would make his life as near perfect as possible so that he could set the goals necessary to reach this ideal. The man began by imagining a life minus things he didn't like. For example, he did not want a repeat of some hardships he had experienced—financial losses, an emotionally draining breakup, a nagging repetitive stress injury—or unpleasant surprises. He banished these banes of daily existence from his imagined world. He also fantasized about a life of greater comfort and material success: money in the bank, good investments, a lovely home. Soon the man had conjured up a detailed vision of a life of ease pleasure and the absence of struggle.

But this man did not stop. He wanted to see how this fantasy might play out over time. With his therapist's help, he forced himself to be intellectually honest. Would his life be interesting and fulfilling without a certain element of surprise or without an occasional struggle or conflict to solve? He had to admit it would not. Gradually this man revised his vision of a dream life and, to his surprise, added back, one by one, most elements he had previously eliminated. The perfect life he imagined was nearly the life he had been living when he began the exercise.

The point? Often people are sure that major obstacles must be *removed* in order for them to progress in making a personal change. But obstacles serve a purpose.

Some are undeniably unpleasant, tough, even heartbreaking, but from the perspective of life as a school, all provide lessons—and opportunities to grow. Without the contrast of surprise, difficulty, and challenge, we would not appreciate pleasures in quite the same way. More than that, we might not acquire the tenacity required to open ourselves and embrace everything life brings us. And we could well miss opportunities to develop emotional stamina, self-control, and that most elusive of all traits: wisdom.

The school of life presents opportunities to learn. Your choices and the quality of your attention determine what you absorb. Your choices are the means by which you play the role of director. You can choose to view your experiences—good and bad, uplifting and disheartening—as opportunities for learning. If you do not, you could wind up snoozing your way through life's curriculum and never finding out what love means, what friendship is, or how insight grows.

Once you see life as a school, there is no need to fight the curriculum. Instead, you can choose to look upon obstacles as opportunities from which to learn and experiences that deepen your understanding of yourself, others, or the world outside you. The school of life is always in session. This day, this week, this month is no exception. What are you learning right now?

FAQ: *Why Don't We Make Changes We Know Are Good for Us?*

Psychologists have puzzled for decades over the question of why people don't make beneficial changes. Some have blamed genetics, character flaws, insufficient knowledge, inadequate discipline, or lack of motivating incentives. Such explanations all apply to certain individuals at certain times. We know from research (our own and others) that at times some people fail on purpose because they don't want to go all out and risk falling short after putting everything on the line. They would rather fail because they did not try. Although they might claim not to care, sadly, they accept less than they secretly want.

More simply and maybe more commonly, people often fail to make a positive change because they don't know the science of how to do so—nor do the health experts who assume that simply repeating messages like "smoking kills" and "just say no" will trigger personal change.

Knowing something is harmful isn't enough to change habits. People fully aware of the grim consequences of smoking continue to puff away. Even personal preferences don't dictate health behavior. Someone who detests the smell and taste of cigarettes may smoke nonetheless. Remember what we told you earlier about defining yourself on the basis of your past experiences? People who smoke usually think of themselves as *smokers*, not of smoking as something they have habitually done. Even when individuals realize they may pay a high price for smoking and think that they should quit, they may not take action. Only when they see a clear way to change do they begin the process.

Think of a healthy change you know you should make but haven't yet. Maybe you don't always buckle your seat belt. Maybe the only vegetables you eat are the mushrooms and onions on a pizza. You already know the benefits of wearing seat belts and eating vegetables. What would it take for you to decide to change?

In a review of 129 studies of behavior change strategies, the individuals who committed themselves to change for positive reasons were the most likely to succeed. Those motivated by a sense of guilt, fear, or regret were less likely to achieve lasting change. Tuck this lesson away. As beings, we move toward pleasure and away from pain. Scolding yourself is a form of self-attack. Stay away from it. Once you choose to change, the skills you will acquire as you read and work your way through *An Invitation to Personal Change* will take you very far in the direction you want to go.

Bad Risks, Good Risks: Knowing the Difference

College is when students want to experiment, enjoy, stretch—and take some risks. But there is a difference between the risk of belting down tequila shooters and the risk of forming a band or trying out for a team. One is a mindless exercise in excess that leaves you with a headache or hangover while the others impart the thrill that comes with daring something new and mastering a challenge. Are you taking risks that don't make sense and that don't add pleasure or passion to your life? Or are you taking risks that empower and inspire you?

Risky behaviors are not new or unusual on campus, but today's students face different—and potentially deadlier—risks than undergraduates did a generation or two ago. Now, as then, many students are sexually active, but these days sexually transmitted infections are more serious and widespread. Despite the dangers, almost three in four students say that they've engaged in unprotected sex at some time—yet somehow most don't feel that they put themselves at risk. (Whether they contracted a disease or not, these students did put themselves at risk.)

Drinking also has long been a part of college life, but nowadays more students drink to excess. Despite efforts across U.S. college campuses to curb alcohol abuse, 4 in 10 undergraduates report having engaged in binge drinking (consumption of five or more drinks in a single session for men, four for women). According to the National Center on Addiction and Substance Abuse, drinking kills an estimated 1,700 students a year and injures more than half a million. Heavy drinking also increases the likelihood of other risky behaviors, including smoking and drug use.

We're not giving you this information to scare you or to preach to you. The problem is not that students who engage in risky behavior are unaware of the danger or that they feel invulnerable. Young people, according to recent research, actually overestimate the risk of some outcomes. However, they overestimate the benefit of the immediate pleasure of taking the risk and underestimate the negative consequences. The ones who do not practice safer sex, for instance, say something like, "This feels too good to stop. Sure, I could get a disease, but how bad is that?" They find out too late.

Here's the bottom line: You do not have to suffer the negative consequences of extreme and unsafe risk taking in order to experience exhilaration and a sense of passion and aliveness. It's your life story and your movie. Observe your experiences closely, and you will see what most people who pay attention discover: Happiness—even excitement—derives from the *process* of fully engaging, of taking on challenges that grow out of big, wild dreams and aspirations. Satisfaction comes from knowing you gave everything you had, not just from achieving certain results. If you get the results you wanted, great. But deep satisfaction does not come from taking risks that unnecessarily threaten your well-being. Love yourself more than that. Treating yourself lovingly is altruistic. As one leader in mindfulness meditation puts it, "Love yourself for everyone else's sake."

We repeat: Watch closely. Pay attention to your life and to your experiences. The lessons are all there. What is working? What is not working? A particular class is over when you learn the lesson it teaches. Are you going to learn quickly or slowly?

The more carefully you pay attention, the more you will see that situations that bring harm often share certain characteristics. They often involve your behaving a certain way to buy some kind of immediate rush or presumed external approval. Yet what looks like approval often does not turn out to be genuine—and you have to live with the consequences of your choices.

Many young people report that when they choose potentially self-harming actions, they override an internal sense of conscience because they want to appear cool, free, or uninhibited. On reflection, they realize that they had magnified out of all proportion the fun they expected and had gained little except regrets.

FAQ: *Don't Most People Who Try to Change Give Up in a Few Months?*

According to various estimates, between 40 and 80 percent of those who try to kick bad health habits lapse back into their unhealthy ways within six weeks. Six weeks, not so incidentally, is about the halfway point for any number of simple and extremely useful changes. In other words, people draw the wrong conclusions from feeling awkward and unsuccessful. On their way to butterflyhood, they quit before they leave the caterpillar stage. Again the culprit is a lack of knowledge.

Successful changers, in contrast, all have one thing in common: they don't give up. In a study of individuals who made New Year's resolutions, two-thirds abandoned their good intentions. But the third who achieved their goals did so in the same way: they kept plugging away for at least six months. By then they had wired their new behavior into their brains. The changes that had seemed so strange and unsettling in January had turned into habits, a normal part of their routine, by July.

It's not unusual to run out of steam on any task, even—perhaps especially—when you're almost finished. In a classic psychology experiment, volunteers repetitively packed then unpacked shoeboxes with small wooden spools. Boring? Crushingly. Monotonous? Beyond belief. When psychologists compared people performing this mind-numbing task for three, six, or nine hours, the results were surprising: No matter how long subjects were assigned to work, all managed to persevere until about the last 15 minutes or so. Then something shifted inside, and they found those last minutes unbearable.

To make sure that you go the distance, plan for and rehearse for longer and more arduous effort and more intense discouragement and disappointment than you could ever possibly encounter. Doing so will provide plenty of energy in reserve when you're tempted to throw in the towel. If you expect it could take 6 weeks to replace a particular habit, prepare to continue for 12 weeks. If you expect your friends to tease you, think of the most disparaging taunts possible and rehearse your pithy retorts or cool silence.

Staying Healthy on Campus

College students generally don't earn good grades for their health habits. Often on their own for the first time, students leave behind their families' ways of eating, sleeping, and relaxing and develop habits and routines of their own. Often they're not healthier ones.

Sleeping less, juggling more, and trying to jam too many things into too few hours, you can quickly end up exhausted—and at greater risk for colds, flu, digestive problems, and other maladies. Freshman year poses the greatest challenge. In national surveys, the majority of freshmen say their daily diet has changed—for the worse. Many put on extra pounds—although generally less than the notorious "freshman 15."

As they log more time in classrooms or at computers, students sit more and move less. Only about a third of undergraduates exercise regularly. The combination of unhealthy eating habits and a sedentary lifestyle can set the stage for a host of medical problems. By the time they graduate, one in four students has at least one major risk factor for diabetes or heart disease.

In the American College Health Association's National College Health Assessment survey, undergraduates rank stress as the number one impediment to academic performance. Sleep difficulties, an epidemic on most campuses, further undermine well-being. More undergraduates are seeking psychological counseling to deal with the strain they feel, as well as for mental disorders such as anxiety and depression. (The *Labs for An Invitation to Personal Change* addresses these issues.)

Yet health problems are not inevitable. You can do more than anyone else to prevent or overcome them because when it comes to your health, you call the shots. No one but you controls what goes in your mouth. You decide which foods to eat, whether to take vitamins, and when to sleep or exercise. You determine when to see a doctor, what kind of doctor, and with what sense of urgency. You decide what to tell the physician and whether to follow his or her advice, take a prescribed medication as directed, or seek further help or a second opinion. The entire process of maintaining or restoring health depends on your decisions. It cannot start or continue without them.

The personal change exercises in the *IPC Labs* offer specific strategies for psychological well-being, stress management, nutrition, fitness, and other dimensions of health. They will be most useful if you keep in mind that lasting change depends not on external rewards but on intrinsic rewards and a sense of achievement. The essential value of what you're doing—the sheer joy of living in a taut, toned body, for instance, or the serenity you gain from daily breathing and meditation practices—is the most powerful incentive.

FAQ: *What If I Blow It?*

Welcome to our club. Failing means you are learning something new. When you couldn't stay up on skates or skis the first time, did you blow it? Or was it just stage one? Failure is essential for change. When you direct a personal change, you make attempts, learn from your mistakes, and gradually refine your skills. Be willing to experiment. Take aim in the right direction, see where you missed and by how much, then take aim again. You must submit to feeling clumsy and to failing if you want to learn.

Setbacks are not only part of the process of change but also evidence that you are changing. When you leave familiar grooves and carve new pathways, you encounter barriers. Even when change goes well, you may briefly revert to older, more familiar behaviors or you may hit plateaus, drift off course, momentarily slide back, then have to right yourself again. Avoid worrying, and don't wring your hands. Setbacks are as ordinary as falling when learning to skate. If you turn them into a big deal, they become a big deal—a justification for quitting.

This does not mean you should complacently accept and repeat setbacks, which are unpleasant and steal time. Do everything in your power to avoid them. The power tools of personal change in Part II of this book can prevent pointless, repetitive setbacks. Otherwise, learn to love your setbacks. Hug them.

Although you do not have control over everything, you do have control over your responses. If you don't find the help you had expected or you run into obstacles you never anticipated, respond with an attitude of acceptance. "Oh, a setback," you might think to yourself. "That's interesting. How did I do that?" Reflect on it and investigate ways to prevent its recurrence. But sometimes all you can say is, "I guess you can't get it right the first time," or "Nobody's perfect." Then move on.

Changing for Good

Whether you see yourself as author of your autobiography or director of your life story, you continuously face choices. Now you face the choice of change. Maybe you're still in the precontemplation or contemplation stages—the two longest phases in the process of change. Or you may be ready to begin the third stage of preparation and to take concrete steps toward your goal.

Wherever you are, you need not remain frozen in this moment, looking over your shoulder, your gaze fixed on the past, always just about to make the choice that will change your life but never quite making it. You have only to turn, face the present moment, and begin to work from your current position. Until you do, you remain mired in what you already know rather than moving ahead to what you have yet to learn. The pain to avoid is knowing what to do but not doing it.

Every day you choose whether and how to express love, creativity, and excellence. Regardless of what you choose, your choices have consequences. Ask yourself: What am I doing with my time? What do I need to do to express who I am? Pick one new thing to do each day that can raise your "standard of living." What is the center point of your life? How do you nurture and nourish your spirit? Are you so busy doing everything that you enjoy nothing?

If you read a few pages from a good book every evening and spend a bit of time thinking about how you want to make tomorrow satisfying, you will begin something you will not want to set aside. If you turn off your iPod or car radio and drive everywhere in silence, you create a noise-free zone—a pagoda for you. Better yet, get out of your car and walk or bike.

You can make better choices. The small decisions of everyday life—what to eat, where to go, when to study—are straightforward. Larger issues—which major to choose, what to do about a dead-end relationship, how to handle an awkward work-study situation—are more challenging. However, if you think of decision making as a process, like change, you can break down even the most difficult choices into manageable steps:

- **Set priorities.** Rather than getting bogged down in details, step back and look at the big picture. What matters most to you? What would you like to accomplish in the next week, month, year? Look at the decisions you're about to make in the context of your values and goals.
- **Inform yourself.** The more you know—about a person, a position, a place, a project—the better you can evaluate it. Gathering information may involve formal research, such as an online search for relevant data, or informal conversations with teachers, counselors, advisers, family members, and friends.

- **Consider all your options.** Most complex decisions don't involve simple either–or alternatives. List as many options as you can, along with the advantages and disadvantages of each.
- **Tune in to your gut feelings.** After you've gathered the facts and analyzed them, listen to your intuition. Although it's not infallible, your sixth sense can provide valuable feedback. If something just doesn't feel right, try to figure out why. Are there fears you haven't confronted yet? Do you have doubts about taking a certain path? "Go with your gut" is not just a pat expression. Researchers have learned that the gut contains neural tissue that is effectively the same as brain cells.
- **Consider a worst-case scenario.** When you're close to a final decision, imagine what will happen if everything goes wrong—the workload becomes overwhelming, your partner betrays your trust, or your expectations turn out to be unrealistic. If you can live with the worst consequences of a decision, you're probably making the right choice.

Fasten your seatbelt. We have made our case for personal change and let you know that it is possible to change more efficiently and easily than you probably imagined. Our intention has been to help you move from precontemplation to contemplation. In the next section you will discover the exhilaration of preparation, action, and locking in gains.

Real change: Tomorrow is another Diet

At age 8, Jessica hoarded candy bars she'd eat late at night. In high school, she'd treat herself to a chocolate shake if she'd blown a test or quarreled with a friend. As the pounds piled on, Jessica tried dieting. Nothing but egg whites and grapefruit one time. Fiber bars and prepackaged meals another. She lost weight. She gained it back. In her senior year, she stuck to a liquid diet for six months. Her mother said she'd never looked better or thinner than on graduation day.

At college Jessica can't seem to avoid overeating. Almost every night she shares takeout pizza to get to know the girls on her floor. She microwaves popcorn when she wants to take a study break. When she's feeling homesick, she devours dishes like pecan pie with whipped cream.

Two weeks ago Jessica finally worked up the courage to step on the scale in the gym. Sure enough, she had put on 6 pounds. She was determined to go on a diet immediately—until her roommate offered her some fudge. "Why not?" she thought. "I'll start tomorrow." Jessica's said the same thing every day since.

To find out what Jessica does—or doesn't do—about her weight, turn to Chapter 11.

Real change: off track?

Hameed knows how lucky he is just to be in college. He knows how much his parents gave up when they immigrated to the United States. He knows the struggles they faced and the sacrifices they made for his sake. He knows how proud they were when he graduated from high school and won a scholarship. And he knows how worried they are that if his grades keep slipping, he won't get into graduate school.

What Hameed doesn't know is why he's foundering now. Sure, his science courses are hard, but no harder than others he's taken. Sure, he's been busy since his roommate talked him into helping with the lighting for drama department productions, but he still studies and hands in assignments on time. So why is he getting Cs instead of his usual As? And why does everyone from his parents to his advisor to his professors seem more upset than he is?

To find out whether Hameed manages to get back on track, see the continuation of this Real Change in Chapter 12.

When you started this book, you may have thought of personal change as frightening, painful, or all but impossible. Now you know better. The formula for real, lasting change is simple: Accept your feelings, know your purpose, and do what you need to do.

You've been on the brink of breakthrough change before. This time we want to take you past the brink. The following exercise can help you move forward.

CLASSROOM ACTIVITY : Your Line in the Sand

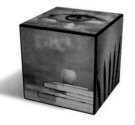

If you do this activity in class, clear a space in the room and draw an imaginary line in the sand. One side of this imaginary line represents life as you have lived it in the past. The other side represents your new life. Crossing the line represents a complete, final, no-turning-back decision to make a change or a series of changes that will help you create the life you want.

Begin by having everyone stand on the side representing the past. Those who have already crossed the line internally or who are ready to do so at this moment should move to the other side. If you have not crossed or you are not ready to cross, position yourself closer or farther from the line, depending on how ready you are.

This is not an exercise in coercion but an assessment done in physical space that relates to crossing an internal line of committing to action. It allows each person in the class to represent physically where he or she is at internally at this moment. No one who is not ready should cross the line. You must do so on your terms, but understand that in order to change you must cross the line at some point. When you do cross, precontemplation and contemplation end and preparation and action begin.

You also can do this exercise on your own. Although you can simply visualize crossing the line, we urge you to do the actual physical exercise. Doing this exercise in space and time adds a powerful, kinesthetic effect that makes the activity far more memorable.

Stand in a room of your choosing and draw an imaginary line in the sand, with one side representing your past life and the other the life that is yours to make. If you have already crossed the line internally or are ready to do so at this moment, step across it physically. Note how you feel. If you have not yet crossed it, choose a position in relation to the line and note how it feels to be where you are now.

Do not make crossing more complicated than it is. All we are talking about is an exercise that testifies to your moving from getting ready to change to taking the actual steps of changing.

JOURNALING ASSIGNMENT : Crossing the Line

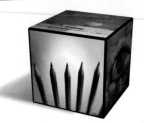

In your *IPC Journal* or in the spaces that follow, write the date and describe where you are in relation to the line. If you have just crossed the line, draw a strong, dark vertical line on the page and record your feelings before you crossed the line and after crossing.

If you have not yet crossed the line, answer the following:

1. How far are you from the line?

_____

_____

_____

_____

2. How ready are you to cross the line?

_____

_____

_____

_____

VISUALIZATION : Crossing the Line

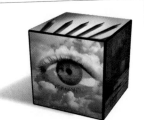

If you have not crossed the line, visualize yourself crossing the line despite not feeling that it is time to do so. Note your response and record your feelings. Then answer the following questions, designed to help you see what preparation you may still need to complete.

1. Is there something that remains in the way of your crossing? If yes, what?

_____

_____

_____

_____

_____

2. If so, are you ready to remove this barrier?

_____

_____

_____

_____

_____

3. If not, when might you be ready to remove it?

_____

_____

_____

_____

_____

4. Is there anything you need to do or find out before crossing?

_____

_____

_____

_____

_____

5. Does further delay bring any advantage? If so, what is it?

_____

_____

_____

_____

_____

6. Is there some other reason to postpone crossing the line?

_____

_____

_____

_____

_____

7.   Is there something more important for you to do first?

_____

_____

_____

_____

_____

After years of study, we have concluded that there is seldom an advantage to deferring change to some future time just to postpone it. Even if it's a stretch, go ahead. Cross the line. By doing so, you go for your change goals now. Whether or not you reach all of them, you head toward a life that will be more interesting and fulfilling.

If, however, there is more you need to know or learn or if some other kind of preparation required, get busy doing it. Then come back to this activity in a week to evaluate your progress in relation to the line. If you have completed all that is necessary, you should find that you are ready to cross to preparation and action.

PART TWO

The Power Tools of Personal Change

Think back to when you first learned how to use a computer—if you can remember. You may have been playing computer games and e-mailing friends for as long as you recall. Depending on your inclination, you may now use your computer for dozens of things, from downloading music to researching papers to paying tuition. But whatever you do, you are constantly employing basic skills you learned long ago.

The power tools in this section function in the same way. They empower you to make successful, lasting personal changes. Once you master them, these practical skills will become automatic and universal. Depending on the situation, either with careful thought or without even thinking, you will apply them in any context to direct any type of change.

Take the time necessary to complete the exercises and assignments in these chapters. Be sure to focus extra effort on ones that seem foreign to your usual way of operating or that might demand an extra stretch to master fully.

For many people, it is easier to talk about a behavior they want to change than to do something about it. As you work your way through this section, just do. Don't think that you need to become something first or fix something external; don't convince yourself that someone else is the problem or is getting in your way. When people make up these kinds of storylines for their personal movies, they delay taking the inevitable needed action.

Don't wait until you feel like doing something before you do it. If you've launched a big project, break it into parts. Make things you want to do convenient to do. Keep tools handy and reminders visible. Make habits you want to eliminate difficult to do. Don't stash candy bars in your desk "just in case" you get hungry. Smoke one cigarette from a pack and throw away the others. Tell others what you are going to do, but make sure they are people who will help hold you to your plan.

Remember that effort equals good fortune. Now let's get going.

CHAPTER 4

Your Personal GPS

41

The global positioning system (GPS), which uses a network of 24 satellites, can pinpoint the location of a car, boat, computer, or cell phone anywhere in the world. Highly accurate, GPS calculates latitude and longitude and tracks movement in any weather conditions, 24 hours a day, seven days a week.

As you move from the contemplation to the preparation stage of personal change, it's time to use your internal GPS to get real. You can't go anywhere new until and unless you know exactly where you are now. Worry about getting to Point B later; first you need to get the coordinates for your personal Point A.

Each of the exercises in the *Labs for An Invitation to Personal Change* begins with a specific "Get Real" self-survey. But before you home in on a single change, get your bearings. Start by asking yourself three key questions. You can write your answers in your *Journal for An Invitation to Personal Change* or here:

1. What am I doing now that I want to stop doing?

    _____

    _____

    _____

    _____

    _____

2. What am I *not* doing now that I want to do?

    _____

    _____

    _____

    _____

    _____

3. What am I doing now that I want to increase or decrease?

    _____

    _____

    _____

    _____

    _____

After you write down your answers, roll them around in your mind. Add, subtract, or edit as your thoughts evolve. These three questions will provide a bird's-eye perspective on where you are now. To zoom in and get a more detailed view, complete the following self-survey.

Where Are You Now?

Self-appraisals help you see where you are already strong and where you need to concentrate your efforts for improvement. The questions that follow provide a basis for a thorough assessment of your strengths and weaknesses.

Write your answers in the space provided or in your *IPC Journal*. Writing forces a different kind of reflection, one more profound than merely saying the answers in your head. Take your time. Think through your responses. Don't judge, rationalize, or blow off any questions. Just be honest with yourself.

Are You Feeling Nervous about Getting Real?

If you are apprehensive about engaging in this kind of self-appraisal, you're in good company. Even the most skilled, most successful, most confident individuals sometimes dread delving into weaknesses—at first. Yet people who achieve important changes learn to embrace self-appraisal because acting on the results of such a candid and personal review gives them a crucial edge in directing change.

Here are four principles to keep in mind as you go through your self-appraisal. They will help keep any anxiety in check:

- **Give yourself balanced feedback.** Every time you finish an answer involving negative traits or something you need to fix, think of qualities that are clearly working for you. This way, you will be less likely to get caught up in focusing only on the negative.
- **Look for the upside.** You'll notice that many negative questions have a corresponding positive one. When you answer a negative question, you might try answering the corresponding positive one.
- **Take your time.** You do not need to complete the entire exercise in one sitting. If you want, take a break or two as you complete the self-appraisal. If you do so, break after answering a positive question so that you finish on a positive note.
- **Stay positive.** If you do start feeling bummed, depressed, or self-critical, shake it off. Engage in another activity for a set amount of time. But before you do, specify when you will come back to work on the appraisal. Be sure to come back to it at this time no matter what.

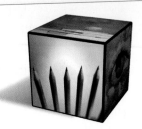

JOURNALING ASSIGNMENT : Assess Yourself

1. Write down a number from 0 to 100 for how you usually feel about yourself. Let 0 represent the worst you could possibly feel about yourself and 100 the best you could possibly feel about yourself.

_____

Circle this number. It stands for how you *usually* feel about yourself.

2. Write down a second number from 0 to 100 for how you feel about yourself *now*. Put the current date beside this number.

_____

3. List what you like about yourself, the qualities that make you feel good about yourself as a person.

_____

_____

_____

_____

_____

_____

_____

_____

_____

_____

4. List what you dislike about yourself, the qualities that make you feel badly about yourself as a person.

_____

_____

_____

_____

_____

_____

_____

_____

_____

_____

5. Write down major assets (such as life experience, a supportive family, special talents, experience living in foreign cultures, or a second or even third language) that you have not yet listed.

_____

_____

_____

_____

_____

_____

_____

_____

_____

6. Write down major limitations (such as financial problems, disabilities, or cultural barriers) that you haven't yet listed.

_____

_____

_____

_____

_____

_____

_____

_____

_____

Test Your Temperament

We all come into the world "wired" with temperamental tendencies. Some of us move toward novel situations, some away. Some resist changes in activity; others are quite adaptable. Some are easily distracted; others lock in like sharpshooters. Different combinations of temperamental qualities provide each of us a baseline as we move into the world. Our environment influences our temperament, and our temperament influences our environment.

The questions that follow allow you to comment on some significant features of your temperament. There are no right or wrong answers. All types of temperament present both advantages and disadvantages, depending on the task at hand.

1. How adaptable are you? Do you go with the flow, or do you resist change?

_____

_____

_____

_____

_____

_____

2. How well do you tolerate frustration?

_____

_____

_____

_____

_____

_____

3. What is your usual mood?

_____

_____

_____

_____

_____

_____

4. Is your energy level high or low?

_____

_____

_____

_____

_____

5. Do you move quickly or slowly toward new situations?

_____

_____

_____

_____

_____

_____

_____

6. Can you concentrate on a task, or are you easily distracted?

_____

_____

_____

_____

_____

_____

_____

Rate Your Master Skills

Remember the master skills we introduced in Chapter 2? Go back to pages 21–24 and read through the descriptions. Then ask yourself the following questions:

1. Are you orderly? When and when not?

_____

_____

_____

_____

_____

_____

_____

_____

2. Do you drop things when they become difficult or less exciting in order to go on to something new? Or do you persist despite obstacles or frustration?

_____

_____

_____

_____

_____

_____

_____

3. Do you work consistently to achieve a goal, or do you work in fits and starts?

_____

_____

_____

_____

_____

_____

_____

4. Have you trained yourself to put in the "reps" (repetitions) needed to acquire a new strength or capacity?

_____

_____

_____

_____

_____

_____

_____

5. Do you complete things you begin?

_____

_____

_____

_____

_____

_____

_____

Know Your Work Style

Because of our different temperaments, talents, and experiences, we develop a work orientation, or a characteristic approach to study and work. Some of us love rolling up our sleeves and digging deeply into a challenge. Others tend to move away from situations that require intensive work.

1. What is your usual attitude toward challenging yourself?

_____

_____

_____

_____

_____

_____

2. Are you self-directed? Do you get going without someone else's prodding?

_____

_____

_____

_____

_____

_____

3. Do you take initiative, or are you passive? When do you take initiative and when not?

_____

_____

_____

_____

_____

_____

4. Are you realistic about what will be required to accomplish tasks?

_____

_____

_____

_____

_____

_____

5. Do you sidestep the essential by getting lost in busywork?

_____

_____

_____

_____

_____

_____

6. Do you skip steps you consider unpleasant?

_____

_____

_____

_____

_____

_____

Appraise Your Fears

If you love tackling work head on, you may not feel fearful or hesitant. But even people with a track record of successes can feel shaky when they move from one level of challenge to another. Although you may have been the best math student in high school, your first college math class may make you question your capacities. Or you may have worked in a shop or made cold calls to potential customers for years yet feel petrified at the prospect of giving an oral class presentation.

At each new life transition we face certain moment-of-truth experiences that can make us wonder whether we have the goods. Although natural, this reaction can sometimes instill fear. How you experience these situations is part of what we want you to examine here. We also want you to look at how you deal with situations that call for increased effort. Remember: There are no right or wrong answers. Just be truthful with yourself.

1. Are you fearful of the demands success will bring?

_____

_____

_____

_____

_____

_____

2. Do you fear not living up to expectations? Your own? Your parents? Your friends?

_____

_____

_____

_____

_____

_____

3. Do you fear failure?

_____

_____

_____

_____

_____

_____

4. Do you fear being ordinary?

_____

_____

_____

_____

_____

_____

5. What frightens you most about going after what you want?

_____

_____

_____

_____

_____

_____

6. What do you fear about acquiring new skills or accomplishments?

_____

_____

_____

_____

_____

_____

7. What do you fear about change?

_____

_____

_____

_____

_____

8. What do you fear about staying the same?

_____

_____

_____

_____

_____

_____

9. How do you deal with fear?

_____

_____

_____

_____

_____

_____

▶ *Bravo!*

Congratulate yourself on getting through one of the toughest exercises in this book! It wasn't so bad, was it? Some people would have quit during this exercise because they were unwilling to look. You didn't quit, you persevered, and you finished. You exercised resolve and used it to your advantage.

In one way or another, as you move along in your life, you will need to repeat briefer or perhaps more exhaustive versions of this soul-searching process in order to stay on track. Each time you look inward and take stock, you will arrive at the answers you need more rapidly.

JOURNALING ASSIGNMENT : Create a Timeline

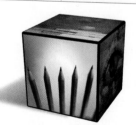

You live in time, and you need a clear sense of time in order to succeed. The following exercise enables you to place the personal change campaign that you're about to launch within the context of your life.

If you are still in the process of identifying your goals and dreams, a timeline may seem premature. Don't worry. You can fill in some parts later. A timeline is part blueprint and part itinerary. As you gather information and use Chapter 8 to formulate your goals, you can make revisions as you see fit.

Think of the timeline at this point as, at best, a rough draft. Use a pencil so that it feels less scary or binding. Remember that the timeline is a guide meant for your benefit alone.

Get a large, poster-sized sheet of paper. On the top half, construct a timeline of your life with an arbitrary life span of 90 years. Mark the events of your life up to the present moment, noting major milestones.

Don't get bogged down. You can approximate dates. Include no more than 10 or 12 major life events (entering kindergarten, your soccer team's regional championship, graduating from high school, and so on). If you have already had a wider range of life experiences than traditional-age college students, you might include your first job, serving in the military, getting married, or having a child. Use words, pictures, photographs—whatever works best for you.

Mark the spot on your timeline that represents today. Based on your self-appraisal and the change you have in mind, mark the date by which you think you will be ready to make your desired change. This is not the same as making a deadline for change; it is a measure of your current sense of when you will be ready to change. Look at your timeline and pencil in the major steps you need to take each day, week, or month to make your desired change.

▶ *Your Secret Power*

If you have a private space for your exclusive use, post your timeline where you can see it daily. If you do not have such a space, put it someplace handy. Keep your timeline away from people who might offer comments and opinions that could derail your progress. Your timeline is about your life and your goals. If someone makes light of your life as it appears on paper, you could use that criticism as a reason to quit before you begin.

A secret has a certain power, a motivating energy. Draw on the secret power of your timeline by reviewing it weekly throughout the term.

Okay. You know where you are. Now you can chart your course.

Real change: clueless on campus (continued)

Alejandra, whom you met on page 12 of Chapter 1, couldn't figure out where to head because she didn't know where she was. Yet the idea of a self-appraisal made her uneasy. What if it she discovered that she wasn't cut out for college? Or that she had chosen the wrong school? It took Alejandra several days to complete the questions in this chapter. As she worked through them, she reflected more on her life and deliberately tried to go deeper and explore her feelings.

For Alejandra, finding her GPS coordinates provided a solid sense of where she was and what she wanted from life. Although she recognized her desire to make her family proud, Alejandra also remembered why she wanted to come to college: She'd always had dreams, big dreams, of discovering a larger world filled with intellectual challenges and exciting opportunities.

As she slowly settled into a routine, Alejandra began to focus on her coursework. Particularly in an introductory anthropology class, she felt a spark ignite inside her brain. The first in her family to be born in the United States, she'd always been curious about her ethnic heritage. Alejandra began to play with the idea of majoring in anthropology and studying different cultures. She particularly loved the idea that her native language, which she hesitated to use with her college friends, would be a great asset in her studies.

As her enthusiasm grew, Alejandra found her attitude toward college shifting. Rather than looking back to what she left behind, she began to look ahead and think about courses to take and study abroad options to investigate. Filled with a sense of a larger purpose, she decided to start volunteering in a community service program. Now firmly planted in her new environment, Alejandra is ready for the next step: developing goals.

Call for Order

Do you live in a state of order? Do you know where your cell phone is right now? Where you put the registration form from student housing? When your geology field project is due? Does it matter? Imagine asking your professor to cut you some slack because you thought the deadline was *next* Tuesday.

Maybe part of you relishes some degree of disorder as testimony to your free spirit, flexibility, or spontaneity. Maybe you think that people who are tidy and organized have less fun. Think again about how you define fun. Is looking for your misplaced student I.D. card or bus pass fun? How about paying late fees at the video store? Every second you hunt for yet another item that's gone missing, every dollar you eventually spend on overdue traffic fines, takes away from the precious time and money you have for yourself. Becoming orderly doesn't take away fun and spontaneity. Instead, it provides the structure and state of mind that make life enjoyable.

Don't assume that some people are just naturally neater or more organized or that you didn't inherit the gene for creating order. Organization is a skill that anyone can learn—fortunately, because disorder steals time. If your goal is to do more than just get by, focus on order. This chapter provides practical strategies and exercises that not only make an immediate difference in your life but also create a solid base for making any personal change.

Sources of Disorder

Disorder arises most often from putting off tasks or not completing an activity you've already begun. The deadly duo of avoidance and postponement multiply the unpleasantness of any chore or assignment. In a matter of days, you face a formidable pile; in a month, you're overwhelmed by an avalanche of routine duties you either haven't started or haven't finished.

Disorder undermines pleasure, as well as efficiency, because it upsets your internal well-being. You need to be in a placid physiological state to feel calm and make good choices. Notice how you feel the next time disorder disrupts your life. Say you can't find the signed medical clearance form you need to join an intramural team. As a result, you have to walk to the farthest corner of the campus and wait who-knows-how-long at the student health service. While madly searching, trudging, waiting, and raging at yourself, you wasted time and energy.

The alternative? Create a solution: an orderly habit that you will *always* follow. Give yourself new operating instructions—in this instance, *always* to put all your important papers in an oversized envelope you *always* keep in the top right-hand corner of your desk.

People vary in how orderly they need their environment to be so that it works for rather than against them. You don't have to become a slave of creating order. However, many college students we know are slaves of disorder. You may pride yourself on being able to roll with the punches that disorder throws at you. But why squander your time cleaning up the consequences of disorder?

Once your physical environment is in order (that is, when you know how and where to put your hands on what you need without delay) you will become more serene and tranquil—in other words, more in order internally. And when you are in internal order, your potential can truly shine.

JOURNALING ASSIGNMENT : One Change at a Time

Identify one problem or hassle caused by a lack of order in your life. Do you, for instance, misplace the class notes you need to study for tests? In your *Journal for An Invitation to Personal Change* or the space that follows, describe the consequences of this specific form of disorder. Then think of one simple change you could make that would prevent or correct it. In this case, you could create a folder for every course and make a habit of putting notes inside after every class. Or you could take class notes in different colored notebooks, one for each class. Try out your solution for three weeks. If you don't see a significant difference, reflect on what you have learned during the three weeks and come up with a more effective modification.

_____

_____

_____

_____

_____

The 15-Minute Clean Up

Who has a whole day to clear out an overstuffed closet or haul months' worth of gear out of the trunk of a car? Of course, you don't. But surely you can snatch 15 minutes from the time you'd otherwise spend surfing the net or watching something forgettable on television. That's all you need to get started.

Don't wait for more disorder to accumulate. And don't fall into the trap of telling yourself that there's no point in starting until you can get it all done at once. You only create more disorder by postponing. Make whatever headway you can in 15 minutes every day during your regular week. On a weekend, set a timer to alert you every hour. Spend 15 minutes organizing and the other 45 minutes however you choose. Before long, you will finish. And if you keep up the same pattern, you will maintain order.

▶ Put Order on Your Calendar

Block out 15-minute slots for targeted bursts of organizational energy on your daily and weekly calendars. Why? Scheduling moves you from "someday, I've got to do this" good intentions (hallmarks of late-stage contemplation and early-stage preparation) to taking action in real time. A schedule, along with specific operating instructions always to follow it strictly, will keep you focused.

Apprentice Yourself

Do you know someone—the grad student in the apartment downstairs, a coworker, a teaching assistant in comparative religions—who always seems organized and on top of things? If so, find a way to take a closer look at that person's habits. Learning how this person stays on top of what once seemed to you to be petty details may provide you with exactly the edge you could use.

Depending on your relationship, you can formally or informally ask this person to share the secrets of the mystery known as order. Ask about the payoffs this person gains from generating order. What it is about order that he or she enjoys? Be curious. Then find out how this person organizes daily life. You may discover pleasure that you never guessed you would find in an orderly life. You certainly will find out that orderly people are not just Goody Two-shoes who tidy up for gold stars.

Seek the counsel of those who keep order because they gain power and find pleasure in devoting immediate attention to things. They may tell you that order not only is useful but also helps create tranquility and control. This inner state of order allows them to do everything else—including their most pleasurable pursuits—with far greater ease. Order ends the constant struggle to overcome disorder, which steals time and inner energy.

Being orderly is a decision. If you hate spending time on meaningless tasks, create a little more order here and a little more order there in every part of your life. Make order an ongoing process. Paying attention to external order creates internal order.

Leave Order Behind

If you don't pay regular attention to the takeout coffee cups piling up on the dresser or the newspapers stacked on the floor, you'll soon find yourself surrounded again by disarray—and feeling out of control. Inattention creates disorder. Sooner or later, you have to tackle the clutter. But if you let disorder become overwhelming, then clearing it becomes an all-out effort that exhausts you. So you slide immediately back into the old approach of not keeping your life in order. Some people repeat this cycle for a lifetime.

Wherever you are—at your desk, on the job, in your room, at home, or in your car—get in the habit of leaving at least one small space more orderly than you found it. This guarantees progress because order becomes an ongoing task, rather than a "once in a blue moon" blitz.

Creating a Workspace That Works for You

You may tell yourself that as long as you have your laptop and wireless access, you can work anywhere—the Student Union, Starbucks, leaning against a tree on the quad, lying in bed in your underwear. You may indeed be able to check a website or send an e-mail, but work—effective, efficient, focused work—requires its own pleasant and well-designed space. You will work best in a space dedicated to a specific activity.

VISUALIZATION : Imagine Your Ideal Workspace

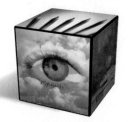

Visualize the place where you can work in your most creative, productive, organized, and energized fashion. What do you see, hear, and feel there? Sense the quality of the light. Feel the air. Smell the smells. How do they induce concentration and encourage you to stay on task? Imagine the furnishings, the colors, and the space that surrounds whatever surface you might use for writing or working at your computer. Picture where and on what you would sit. Make everything perfect for you.

Now imagine how close you can come to creating this space where you live now. What would you have to do to create a place conducive to good work? Given your current budget, how closely can you approximate your ideal environment? When you have finished, make some notes. Then go to work on your workspace.

Here are our recommendations. Use them, along with your visualization and notes.

Ideally, set aside a space for your exclusive use. It should be a private sanctuary that others do not enter. If it's not possible to keep your workstation behind locked doors, ask the people you live with to respect this space and not touch or move the things you leave there. If you reserve one area solely for academics, every time you approach it, your mind will make unconscious associations that provide cues to help you focus on your studies.

Order demands that you have everything ready and at hand. Consider the minimum requirements. For sure, you will need a good-sized flat surface and supplies within easy reach. Think of it this way: Everything in your space should work for you and support you; nothing should work against you. Remove anything that might distract you—telephone, MP3 player, PlayStation, and all photos of your family, your true love, your pet dog, or models with tight abs.

As much as possible, seek good natural and artificial light so that you can work without straining your eyes and adding unnecessary fatigue. Set up your computer to keep glare and eyestrain to a minimum. Make sure you have a good, back-friendly chair and that your desk or table is the proper height.

Arrange the entire environment to convey a simple message: This is a great, comfortable workspace where I rule. Your workspace will work better if it appeals to you aesthetically and beckons you to come and work. Even in a dorm room, surround yourself with your favorite colors. Over time, add small touches to get as close as possible to the most ideal workspace you can imagine.

59

▶ *Don't Hit the Sack*

You've finally finished your last assignment, and you're absolutely, utterly exhausted. You look at the books stacked on the floor and the papers strewn over your desk. "Forget it," you think. All you want to do is crawl into bed. Don't. Take 10 or 15 minutes to put your workspace back in order. Gather the notes for your term paper into a file. Put your textbooks back on the shelf. Taking the time to put your workspace in order produces many benefits, including creating an inviting space to which to return. You'll love yourself even more in the morning.

"What's that weird smell?"

That question—asked by a cute girl Noah, whom you read about on page 26 of Chapter 2, had invited to his room—left him speechless. Mortified, he realized that he hadn't changed the sheets his Mom had put on his bed the day he moved into the dorm. Noah couldn't count how many hamburger wrappers and greasy French fry bags he must have kicked under his desk. And who could guess whether his athletic shoes, socks, or jersey smelled worst?

The next day, Noah bought oversized trash bags and began excavating his room. As a little joke, some friends posted a sign that said, "Danger: Hazardous Waste!" But after hauling out the garbage and doing laundry, Noah still didn't know what to do with his piles of books, papers, and clothes. Wandering down the hall, he stopped by a room that, although no bigger than any other, seemed more spacious. He took note of the file cabinet in the corner, the bookshelves lining one wall, the plastic crates neatly stacked in the closet. When his dormmate told him he'd bought them at a discount office supply store just off campus, Noah headed out to pick up some basic organizers.

Noah loved the new workspace and storage units he set up—until midterms, when a sea of notes, practice tests, texts, clothes, soda cans, and empty chips bags again engulfed his room. After another cleaning marathon, Noah made a vow to spend some time every day on clutter control—although often he got too tired or distracted to bother with putting away stuff.

When Noah joined the swim team, he finally bought himself a daily organizer, just like the ones his teammates used, to keep track of practice times and meets. As his final task every day, he scheduled tidying time and didn't go to bed until he crossed it off his list. Although no one will ever consider Noah a neatnik, he no longer feels that his time and things are beyond control. And his room smells a whole lot less like a pig ranch.

Time Control

Most students struggle to cram all they need and want to do into their busy lives. There's no way around it: Time is a given, and everybody gets the same amount. No one can add a 25th hour to the day or an eighth day to the week. But you can take control of how you use time—even if you think you will always feel out of control. What you choose to do with the time you have is what matters.

This chapter provides step-by-step techniques that will enable you to pay exquisite attention to time and to choose wisely how you use it. As you adopt these strategies, you will accomplish more and will waste less time making up for what you should have done days or weeks ago—or redoing the task you started but did not finish. You may be surprised by how your perspective on time changes. Rather than viewing time as thief or taskmaster, you will celebrate your skill at filling it with things you enjoy.

Becoming conscious of time and how you use it is the crucial first step to taking control of your life. If you want to be planted securely in the director's chair, get on top of your time. Step one is to get real about how you are currently using time.

Your Three-Day Time Diary

Using your *Journal for An Invitation to Personal Change* or the form that follows, keep a log of how you spend you time over a period that includes at least one weekend day. Set a timer—a watch, cell phone, computer, or clock—to go off every 15 minutes and record at that time or as soon as possible what you were doing when the alarm went off.

6:15 a.m.	_____	1:15 p.m.	_____
6:30 a.m.	_____	1:30 p.m.	_____
6:45 a.m.	_____	1:45 p.m.	_____
7:00 a.m.	_____	2:00 p.m.	_____
7:15 a.m.	_____	2:15 p.m.	_____
7:30 a.m.	_____	2:30 p.m.	_____
7:45 a.m.	_____	2:45 p.m.	_____
8:00 a.m.	_____	3:00 p.m.	_____
8:15 a.m.	_____	3:15 p.m.	_____
8:30 a.m.	_____	3:30 p.m.	_____
8:45 a.m.	_____	3:45 p.m.	_____
9:00 a.m.	_____	4:00 p.m.	_____
9:15 a.m.	_____	4:15 p.m.	_____
9:30 a.m.	_____	4:30 p.m.	_____
9:45 a.m.	_____	4:45 p.m.	_____
10:00 a.m.	_____	5:00 p.m.	_____
10:15 a.m.	_____	5:15 p.m.	_____
10:30 a.m.	_____	5:30 p.m.	_____
10:45 a.m.	_____	5:45 p.m.	_____
11:00 a.m.	_____	6:00 p.m.	_____
11:15 a.m.	_____	6:15 p.m.	_____
11:30 a.m.	_____	6:30 p.m.	_____
11:45 a.m.	_____	6:45 p.m.	_____
12:00 p.m.	_____	7:00 p.m.	_____
12:15 p.m.	_____	7:15 p.m.	_____
12:30 p.m.	_____	7:30 p.m.	_____
12:45 p.m.	_____	7:45 p.m.	_____
1:00 p.m.	_____	8:00 p.m.	_____

► *Take a Power Break*

Literally stop and take five. Stretch. Erase all thoughts. Albert Einstein used to lean back in his chair with his keys in his hand. He'd close his eyes, clear his mind of thoughts, and allow himself to relax deeply. The sound of the keys slipping from his hand and hitting the floor would rouse him to go back to work. Try pulling an Einstein. Shift your brain to neutral occasionally.

Dissect Your Day

If you don't analyze where your time is going, you're likely to continue to lose it (or not use it) the same way you always have. Your three-day diary can give you an objective sense of what you chose to do with time over a short period. Use colored highlighters to shade time spent asleep, online, in class, working, studying, getting to and from class, eating, doing chores, e-mailing, talking with friends, and so on. Look for patterns. Calculate the number of hours you spent on various activities.

JOURNALING ASSIGNMENT : Build Pleasure into Your Day

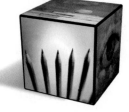

As you record where your time goes, put a plus sign next to those activities that energized or excited you and a minus sign next to those that drained you. Use the data from your recent past to plan your future and put more "pluses" on your calendar. They don't have to be major splurges.

Use your journal to identify positive practices you can weave into your daily routine, such as listening to a playlist of music that stirs or soothes you or looking at the night sky. Once you expose yourself to just a little pleasure, you want more of it. And you can get it. You don't have to wait for the big birthday cake of a vacation; take little bites of cupcake throughout the day every day.

When you take a break, really take one. Switch gears completely. Relax deeply. Unwind in real time with no screen in front of you. Melt into a sofa or hammock. Lie down on a futon. Zone out in a warm bath or hot tub. Let go. Develop a routine that cues relaxation and practice it when you need to relax deeply. Before bed, for instance, clear your mind of thoughts or read for pleasure before you repeat affirmations or review your day and its successes.

Preempting Procrastination

We've all put off until tomorrow things that we would rather not face today—and come up with millions of excuses for procrastinating. There are only two fundamental reasons we do not complete tasks in a timely way: We either lack smart, effective strategies and skills for making efficient use of time, or we fall back on truly inefficient, self-defeating habits that steal precious time. In other words, either you have failed to develop good habits that you need to learn, or you have developed bad habits you need to unlearn and replace. (The "Do It Now" lab in the *Labs for An Invitation to Personal Change* can provide help and practice.)

Most delay springs from fear. People are afraid that they lack the knowledge they'll need to navigate a situation or that their efforts won't succeed. Hesitant to face something they mildly dread, they postpone a report, a phone call, or a delicate conversation; lose time; and increase their dread. This may have happened to you. Unless you immediately research how to handle a situation more effectively, setting something aside instead of acting on it seldom offers an advantage. And you squander time you can never regain.

Start now. Decide what you are going to do for the rest of the day and tomorrow, what will be your top priority, and how you will go about getting your work done. Write down the specific tasks you will complete by the end of the day. Some will be simple chores, like buying shampoo and toothpaste; others will be steps in a larger, ongoing project.

Set your alarm a little earlier than usual. This does not mean you have to get up at 5:00 a.m.—just early enough to start the day in a state of calm contemplation. Don't rush out choking down a doughnut and already running 10 minutes behind. People who get up a half hour to an hour earlier than they once did report amazing changes in their sense of command and their productivity. When your alarm goes off, get out of bed immediately. Welcome the day. When you rise up shining, you set the tone for everything that follows.

Get to your first class or appointment a little before you have to be there. An early arrival sends a message that what you are about to do is significant and not just another throwaway experience to rush through. Just do it and see the difference.

► Begin

The single most effective antidote to procrastination is starting. Don't flog yourself to tackle the chore you hate most; just do step one. If the long-delayed job is cleaning the bathroom, tell yourself that all you are going to do now is take the basic equipment—cleaning solutions, brushes, rubber gloves, whatever—into the bathroom. Once you get there, having started the process, you will find it easier to follow the now imperative and will go ahead and complete the job.

The Now Imperative

"Just do it" is the famous Nike slogan. We would add one more word: just do it *now*. Act the moment a need arises. When you do, you act far more efficiently than when you delay.

The "now" part of this phrase has to do with the optimum time to act. The "imperative" part means there is no other way out. Nothing is as efficient as acting the moment a day-to-day need appears. When you set this standard and adhere to this imperative, you will quickly feel different about yourself and your capacities.

Whenever possible—and it is possible much of the time with a small amount of additional effort—dispatch simple things in one fell swoop. Don't pointlessly break a task down into a series of steps if they aren't necessary. Skip the list-building busywork. Cut directly to the chase. (See the "Do It Now" lab of the *IPC Labs* for more on overcoming procrastination.)

No More Multitasking

As you read this, are you glancing at a text message, scrolling through e-mails, listening to music, or thinking ahead to the weekend? Maybe you're trying to multitask and do all of these at once. Stop! The brain, as neuroscientists have demonstrated, performs even simple actions one after another, in a strict linear sequence. Unless they are completely mechanical activities, multitasking destroys the quality of attention given to the tasks at hand.

So work when you work, play when you play. And talk on your cell phone only when you're doing nothing more important than picking laundry lint off a black T-shirt but never when you're driving.

Turn off your text message and e-mail alerts when you block out 45 minutes for reading your econ assignment. Don't cringe, don't whine; just do what needs doing. Become formidable in your devotion to this habit, and you will have more time for what's really important. When you are finished or ready for a break, you can go back to the text messages. They won't vanish while you are working.

Live in Real Time

Everyone loves a shortcut. In your hometown, do you know the best route to take from Point A to Point B, even in rush hour? Shortcuts make sense only when they enhance true efficiency, not when they simply skip necessary steps. When it comes to time control, the ideal shortcut is acting in real time.

Doing things immediately skips unnecessary steps and requires less effort than doing them later. Many people fail to notice something subtler: Delaying anything is procrastination on a smaller scale. Cumulatively, the consequences are the same: a serious loss of time that, if used well, could have yielded a sense of satisfaction, ease, and control. Instead, when you feel rushed and panicky, your performance is weaker than it might have been.

Say you have to lead a discussion in your political science class. You decide that in order to prepare you need to download a file and look something up in your textbook. You can take the time to jot yourself a note, then add these items to a to-do list. Why? You're engaging in needless delay. Or you can download the file then and there and look up the information in your textbook. This is living in real time.

The people who accomplish the most in the most efficient manner invariably handle these tasks immediately, as they arise. They manage the day-to-day part of their lives now, in real time, not later after a series of pointless delays. The time you spend delaying is the time in which you could have done what you delay. If you learn to respond immediately to ordinary tasks—e-mail, snail mail, calls you need to make—or anything else that you could finish in three minutes or less, you will learn a simple secret that will exponentially increase your efficiency. Just don't interrupt your study time to do them.

Why put your coat on the bed when you can hang it up? Why not forward the announcement of tryouts the first time your friend asks for it? Will staring several times at the button that you need to sew back on a jacket make it easier when you finally get around to doing it a month later? Will waiting to do laundry when you "have time" put a clean sweatshirt that doesn't smell funky in your closet?

You neither have to nor should answer the phone, floss your teeth, put the soup in the microwave, and download a course syllabus at the same time. But if you are not going to complete an action right away, you must *in real time* take the next step required. For instance, if you cannot complete a task in three minutes, you can write it down on a to-do list. But if you never look at the list again, keep several lists in separate places, or scribble reminders on napkins from the cafeteria and stash them in your purse or pocket, writing down what you need to do only wastes time.

Putting off programming your PDA or learning how to use new software is the same. You compound a problem you invested time and money to solve. All alternatives to living and acting in real time create inefficiency. These can range from a minor time loss that drags on resources to, in the worst case, a feeling of being chronically overwhelmed and unable to catch up. Don't buy gadgets and equipment you don't have time to figure out how to use. Learn to use the time-saving, life-brightening devices you already have—like your brain and your attention. Don't put it off any longer. Do it now.

To live in real time does not mean that you assume the ready–fire–aim mode. Rather, instead of setting things aside, respond when they first come to your attention. Acting in this fashion does not rule out considering your actions as thoroughly as warranted. And it does not rule out choosing the best time to do something later if it will take longer than three minutes. *But you must choose the specific time and act when it arrives.* If you need to consult or consider, by all means do so. But don't put this off either. Begin it now, carry through on it as far as possible, and then continue it at a time you choose and record. Do not set aside what you can do now.

Don't Be Derailed by Distractions

Five minutes after you sit down to study, are you checking a price on eBay or downloading a podcast? Foraging for a drink or snack? Turning up your music to blot out your roommate's? If so, stop everything. The external interruptions Ralph Waldo Emerson called "idle distractions" are undermining the messages you need to communicate to your brain about urgency and efficiency.

To stay on track, schedule your work in 55-minute segments, with 5-minute breaks between sessions. Start by taking a few moments to focus and visualize what you're about to do. Turn off your cell phone. Shut off all music; stop fiddling with the wallpaper on your computer screen. Use earplugs if necessary (not earbuds) to block out noise. Build in downtime ahead of time, and take it according to schedule. Keep working at this pace until you complete what you set out to do. You send yourself an empowering message when you keep your promises to yourself.

Rehearsing Real Life

Before you begin a task, whether it's studying statistics or making a timeline for Western Civ, take a few moments to visualize yourself completing the steps the process requires. This cues the mind in another way and prepares it like any other run-through or rehearsal. Why do sports teams practice plays? In fact, why does anyone rehearse anything? Because you perform better when you rehearse. Rehearsal provides a mind map—an internal set of expectations and directions—and serves as a fundamental way of getting ready for peak performance.

This process is also a mental focusing device. All the tugging, wiggling, spitting, and scratching that athletes engage in between pitches or tennis serves is not superstition. This chain of behaviors cues the mind and senses to a keen degree of focused readiness. If you visualize steps, you prepare yourself for action. As research demonstrates, this practice is a big aid to completing things on time.

Develop your own routine to cue yourself that it is time to work. Visualize. Follow a sequence of steps. Work with a sense of urgency. There is a time for leisure and a time for heightened attention and readiness. If you are working on a task, make it a matter of urgency, and you will move toward it differently. This is not about hurry but about force of *intention* and focus of *attention*. Do things deliberately but with a concentrated sense of urgency.

If you have many tasks, do the most difficult ones early in the day. Save the easy ones for the afternoon, when your circadian rhythms dip and your energy lags. Resist the notion that handling the easy ones will provide a sense of accomplishment. Your brain will read that for what it is: avoidance of the difficult things. When you come back to anything you have put off, you always resist it more. Do it first. Then notice how empowered you feel. The rest of the day will accelerate, and your confidence will soar.

Time Control for Commuting and Working Students

If you commute to campus, you can't roll out of bed 10 minutes before class, zip up your jeans, and sprint across the quad. If you work, you have to show up on time, do your job, and fit in studying when and where they can. If you don't take control of your time, you will soon feel out of control.

To beat the time crunch, begin before the term starts. Get the course catalog as early as possible so that you can plan your work hours or commute around it. Try to avoid rush hour traffic or crowded subway trains. Whenever you can, schedule classes back to back or during one part of the day (all morning or all evening, for example) so that you can concentrate academics in one block of time.

Get a calendar, and use it from the first day of the term. This will be your most valuable time control tool. Read the syllabus from each course thoroughly the first day of class. Don't delay, or you will lose valuable time. Mark down on your calendar all assignment due dates and exams. (If an assignment doesn't have a due date, give it one). For any research projects or group assignments, make a schedule on your calendar for how you'll complete each of them. Include "begin research for anthro paper" on one day, "complete outline" a week later, and "begin first draft" on another day.

Breaking big projects up into smaller pieces and giving yourself deadlines for each will help you stay on track. Calculate roughly how many hours you think each assignment will take. (Remember: Most things take longer than you think, so build in extra time from the start.)

Let your professors know your work schedule, and let your boss know your class schedule. Although you cannot expect them to plan around you, they may be flexible with you on due dates and work hours if they know your time demands.

Write Now

People can operate for years or forever under the illusion that writing takes a long time. It does so only because they set aside a lot of time to do it. As a result, the project expands to fill the amount of time they allot. Large chunks of your supposed writing time then involve staring, fidgeting, feeling sorry for yourself, and not writing. Because you predict a battle, you must have one. When it's time to begin writing, do you ever find yourself in the bathroom surveying the Vesuvius-sized pimple that has suddenly erupted on your face?

Problem? You have not set a sufficiently demanding time limit to keep yourself interested. Result? Your mind wanders, and your time escapes. The next time you're assigned a paper, write down the instructor's deadline for turning it in. Then set your own deadline. Make it as soon as possible and stick to it. When you do, indulge your well-earned impulse to strut, but also enjoy the feelings you've created of mastery and internal tranquility. Then, use the time thereafter until the actual due date to polish and refine your paper without feeling stressed. Take note of the difference in your attitude—and in your grade.

JOURNALING ASSIGNMENT : Practice Real-Time Writing

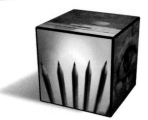

As soon as you read through this assignment, start writing in the space that follows. Describe your typical attitude and approach to writing. Did a term paper ever seem interminable? Did you ever put off starting a paper until you had no choice but to pull an all-nighter? What was the experience like? Did it induce a creative high, or did you freak?

_____

_____

_____

_____

_____

_____

_____

_____

_____

_____

_____

_____

_____

_____

_____

_____

_____

_____

_____

_____

_____

_____

_____

_____

_____

_____

_____

_____

Pause and think: Is there an e-mail you've put off answering or a report you've left on hold? Imagine how you'd feel if you dispatched it immediately. Do it. Write it now.

Learning the Language of Change

Every day we unconsciously hypnotize ourselves with the words we use, when we talk both to ourselves and to others. Depending on their nature, we transmit messages that can paralyze or inspire, mire us down or move us forward. What we say and the words we choose reveal what we believe, expect, and intend. Our language reflects our reality, especially our sense of what we consider possible. Language expresses the expectations we have and the limits we see.

The way you use language either helps keep you stuck where you are or aids in your quest for personal change. You can increase your effectiveness by using language that supports change. Pay attention both to *what* you say and think and *how* you say and think it. Then consciously consider the words in your mind and your mouth. Do they need some editing? What are you telling yourself? This chapter shows you how to choose and use the words that can best help you direct change.

Loophole Language

Are you "trying" to get organized? If so, you've just tripped over your own feet. *Try,* as in "try to do it if you can," is a sorry, sickly little word that insinuates itself regularly into otherwise reasonable requests and kills their power. "I'll try" in response to a request is usually a polite form of refusal. If your professor gives you a date and time to discuss your final grade, would you "try" to make it? This use of *try* differs from the *try* that means to "test or examine."

The word *try,* meaning "to attempt," is a weasel word that contains a built-in implicit directive to stop short of succeeding. When someone says, "just try your best," isn't that person suggesting that you mount some kind of effort but not expect to be successful? To comply fully with the directive "just try your best," you *have* to stop short of bringing something to a successful conclusion. The *just* tells you how far to go. "Try your best" is the same as "Don't worry. I don't expect you to make it."

Think for a moment. Would "try your best" be what you would say to a heart surgeon before going under the knife? The effect of "try to" is the same when you say it to yourself. Soft language, with its built-in slack, gives you and others permission to accept less than your best. When you talk to yourself in this kind of loophole language, you listen to, and follow, the implied directives.

Language that expresses unequivocal intention sounds different and makes different demands on the listener. With it, you create an internal environment of clear objectives and directives. For example, if you say about your zoology final, "I'm gonna try to study hard for it," the word *try* sends a message to your brain that cancels out the "study hard for it." But if you say "I am going to make sure that I ace it," the language requires a different kind of commitment. That's what we're talking about.

People also sabotage themselves by saying "if" or "if only." You probably have used phrases like "If I could get organized" or "If only I could stick with my exercise plan." Such statements reinforce the notion that you're never going to change. Instead of another "if," say to yourself, "When I get organized" or "When I start working out." This simple switch sets the stage for believing what is true—that you already can and will be able to change your lifestyle.

Another way to prevent dodging change is to use the word *how* rather than *why* to explain your actions. For example, if you ask yourself *why* you sometimes drink too much, you might answer, "Things aren't going well in my life" or "I get bored in the evening." If you ask yourself *how* you drink too much, you might answer, "I start playing drinking games with my friends" or "I don't keep track of how many beers I have."

Give yourself new operating instructions and insist that you always follow them. Tell yourself that whenever you reach for another drink, you will always consider how you are choosing or deciding to drink more rather than answering the why question with another excuse for doing so. When you ask how, know that you have a basis for how you choose to drink more.

▶ Don't Try

Forbid yourself for one week from using the word *try* in relation to actions you are going to take. Observe the effect. You will quickly discover how often you use the word—and perhaps why you use it. You will also discover how different it feels to shed this linguistic hideout. You may feel that you are eavesdropping on your own unconscious. Also note how different it is to forbid yourself to use the word than it is to try not to use it.

Straight Talk

If your instructor asked if you'd like to get an A in this course, would you say, "sort of" or "kind of"? We hope not. Vague language invites you to hold back, especially when you're talking about what you want to do. Add "really" to the mix, and you dilute what you're saying even more.

What does it mean to say, "I sort of really want to do it"? This kind of speech carries an ambivalence virus that infects your thinking and your ability to move on things. When you speak of goals, use definitive, unequivocal language to describe what you want and how you intend to get it. Say, "I will do it"—with no "kind of," "sort of" vagueness attached or implied. Notice the difference from the wishy-washy conditional tense and passive voice of "I would like it to get done today." These statements sound different because they are different.

When you start a sentence with "it" or use the passive voice, you suggest that things happen independent of your will or because of external events not under your direction. Compare the differences between the following:

▌ "It needs to get done."
▌ "I need to do it."
▌ "I am doing it today."

All three express differences in locus of control and intention to complete the action. Although you are not in control of everything, the first statement suggests that there is no point in exercising the power you do have and thus excuses you from responsibility. The second statement talks about a need. There is no stated intention and no directive to complete. The difference between the first and the third is night and day in terms or urgency and intention to complete the task at hand.

Ducking responsibility, however appealing at the moment, always costs you heavily. When you linguistically evade responsibility, you reduce personal power and control and invite the passivity that the passive voice implies. Although we're not teaching a grammar lesson, we hope you get the message. By taking greater responsibility *for* your language and *with* your language, you demand that you take greater responsibility *for* your actions and *with* your life. Remember chance versus skill instructions? This is a semantic case in point.

Look for ways to embrace and increase responsibility when you talk. Using the active voice—I am, I do, I will—frees you to seek ways in which you can exert a directing force upon your life. When you use the active voice and embrace as much responsibility for your actions as you can, you will notice a greater sense of mastery and personal efficacy.

Say "I am writing the essay this afternoon." Then do it. Do not say, "I'm going to take a stab at that essay today or tonight—whenever I can get to it." Deconstruct the second sentence, and you will easily recognize how vague your operating instructions are. The odds of your finishing it this afternoon by saying it the second way are next to nothing. Why? Because you didn't say anything that remotely expresses this specific intention and because the instructions to your brain are vague. To follow those vague instructions, your brain actually has to take vague actions and not complete the task. In plain language, you aren't planning to, so you won't.

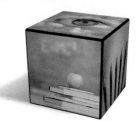

CLASSROOM ACTIVITY : Talk the Talk

Write a dialogue involving at least six exchanges between two characters discussing a task or assignment. Write in the passive voice with vague specifications, such as "sort of," "kind of," and the deadly phrase "will try." Get together with another student and jointly revise each other's dialogues so that they express clear, unequivocal intention and personal responsibility for completing the task.

Read both versions in front of the class. Be dramatic. Have fun, and in the process notice how different language makes you feel and act differently. Ask your audience members which version they think would be more likely to lead to action.

No More Negatives

Eavesdrop on what you say to others and to yourself in the course of a day. When you do, listen for limiting statements, such as "I hate exercise" or "I can't learn calculus." Such comments keep you stuck where you are—and feeling bad about yourself. They also severely limit your sense of personal efficacy.

You can talk your way out of self-limiting statements. Instead of saying, "I hate exercise," say, "I am learning to enjoy exercise" or "I choose to like exercise." Instead of "I can't learn calculus," switch to "I haven't learned calculus *yet*." Hear and feel the difference. Reversing negative statements is a gentle but effective tool that increases your awareness of possibilities and changes your supposed limits.

If you are in a situation in which you cannot or do not wish to reverse a negative statement aloud (in a classroom, for instance), you can do it in your head. An alternative way to cancel out the negative statement is to say to yourself "delete" or "cancel" as quickly as possible following the statement.

When you talk about a negative behavior, trade the present for the past tense. If you think "I'm selfish," switch to "I used to be selfish in the past." Change a statement such as "I always get excited about starting something new but then get discouraged and quit" to "I used to get excited about starting something new but then got discouraged and quit."

When you move negative habits or characteristics into the past, you stop hanging on to them. Changing the tense helps you differentiate between what you did in the past and what is possible now. You remind yourself that you have changed, are changing, or at least are capable of change.

In your *Journal for An Invitation to Personal Change* or in the space that follows, make a list of some positive attributes you plan to acquire. If you'd like to be assertive, confident, and self-assured, claim these characteristics as your own now. Write a series of statements describing the new, improved you—all in the present tense. Using the present tense creates a hypnotic-like demand that your behavior match the description—the very reason that we want you to talk about negative characteristics in the past tense.

JOURNALING ASSIGNMENT : What Do You Choose?

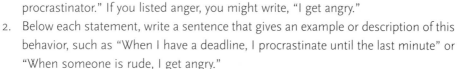

1. In your *IPC Journal,* go back to the list of negative or limiting attributes you compiled in Chapter 4. Take five of these characteristics, and make a simple, self-descriptive statement with each one. For example, if you listed "procrastination," you might write, "I am a procrastinator." If you listed anger, you might write, "I get angry."

2. Below each statement, write a sentence that gives an example or description of this behavior, such as "When I have a deadline, I procrastinate until the last minute" or "When someone is rude, I get angry."

3. Next, directly below each sentence, rewrite it, inserting the word *choose.* For example, you would write, "When I have a deadline, I choose to procrastinate until the last minute" or "When someone is rude, I choose to get angry,"

4. Now rewrite each sentence again, making the following significant change: Put the sentence in the past tense and modify it with an adverb, like *often,* that acknowledges you have not always behaved in the same way. For instance, you could write, "When I've had deadlines in the past, I often used to choose to procrastinate until the last minute" or "When someone has been rude, I sometimes used to choose to be angry."

5. When you have completed the preceding steps, reread all forms of the sentences you have written, noticing the difference each simple change makes in the way you experience choice and the possibility for change. Introducing a key word, a change in tense, or a simple modifier makes each sentence reflect a progressively less limiting idea of reality and more accurately acknowledges your freedom to choose. You are not bound by your past choices unless you decide to be. Understand and feel the difference as you read each sentence.

6. Now take this exercise to a new level: In the space below the last sentence you wrote, write a sentence about a new positive behavior. For example, you might write, "When I have a deadline, I work in a timely way" or "When someone is rude, I don't take it personally or allow myself to get angry."

7. After you complete the new positive alternative sentence, take another long look at each item and the sentences you have written below it. Let the progression sink in.

8. For two full weeks, repeat the new final sentence you have written five times upon rising and five times before sleeping. It is crucial that you complete this step, because it lays down a new internal format, a new thought platform from which you can operate. As you change your internal dialogue, you create an association between yourself and this new quality.

Don't Skip a Step

Once you have a sense of the word changes involved in this exercise, you may be tempted to create the new sentences only in your mind. Resist. You must rewrite each statement with each modification. You will miss out on crucial benefits if you skip any of these steps.

Talk to Yourself

"Every day, in every way, I'm getting better and better."

You may have heard this phrase so often that you dismiss it as a cliché of pop feel-good psychology. It's not.

In the early 1920s Emile Coué, a French therapist, developed a technique called *conscious autosuggestion,* which required repeating this phrase 20 times on awakening and 20 times before retiring. Through the years, researchers around the world have confirmed that repeating a positive statement affects self-perceptions and self-esteem. Frequent repetition of an affirmation, a motivating phrase or sentence, has become a fundamental part of cognitive-behavior therapy.

When you are working on personal change, saying an affirmation over and over in your head is one of the fastest ways to restructure your thought patterns, develop new pathways in your brain, and change your mindset. Try one of the following:

- "I am responsible for my life choices, and I allow others to be responsible for theirs."
- "I take charge of my choices and complete what is required to reach my goals."
- "I take an active role in directing change in my life toward a healthier, happier me."

If none of these affirmations suits you, make up one of your own. Make your affirmation positive, use the present tense, and target the change you desire. Write down your affirmation, and be sure to make the phrase as clear and compelling as possible. Then say it to yourself.

How often? You'll need to repeat your affirmation at least five times in the morning when you arise and in the evening just before going to sleep. More is better, however. If you want, add an emotionally positive image that summarizes the realization of the affirmation after the five repetitions. Say your affirmation while doing any simple task—taking a shower, brushing your teeth, gelling your hair, sitting in traffic, emptying the dishwasher, walking to the bus stop, riding an elevator, or waiting for your computer to boot.

Although you aren't conscious of what is happening, your affirmation will create a new pathway of connections in your brain. Within a short time, you'll find that you no longer use the old habitual thought you've forsaken. As you keep repeating your affirmation, you'll feel a greater desire to stick with your new behavior.

JOURNALING ASSIGNMENT : Just Because

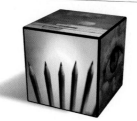

According to social psychology research, using the word *because* when making a request or seeking agreement can boost your compliance as high as 80 to 90 percent. Even when you talk to yourself, using the word *because* shifts your brain to a deeper level of analysis. For instance, you might tell yourself the following:

"I eat more fruit because I want to eat more nutritiously."

"I do some form of exercise each day because I want to be strong and flexible."

"I meditate because I want to lower my stress level."

Now it's your turn. In your *IPC Journal* or the space below, jot new sentences that follow the preceding pattern.

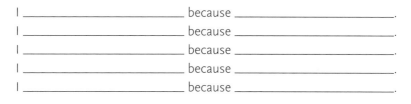

I _____ because _____.
I _____ because _____.
I _____ because _____.
I _____ because _____.
I _____ because _____.

▶ *Nod Your Head*

Social psychologists have discovered that when you nod your head yes while you repeat something you accept, you significantly strengthen your acceptance of, belief in, and likelihood to follow what you are saying. Ready for an experiment? (Nod your head yes!)

Go back and reread the paragraphs in this section. Nod your head yes as you do so. You might do the same throughout each chapter that follows. Every time a new significant idea is mentioned that you want to absorb and follow, nod your head yes. Just because.

CHAPTER 8

Going for Your Goals

Your Big Picture

Be Specific ◄

Journaling Assignment: Dream Big

Visualization: See Your Dream

Ask the Big-Picture Questions ◄

Your Master Plan for Getting to Your Goals and Dreams

Classroom Activity: Share Your Master Plan

Become a Goal-Getter

Owning Your Goals ◄

Journaling Assignment: Setting Long-Term Goals

Setting Short-Term Goals

Don't Settle for Halfway ◄

Real Change: Second Time Around (continued)

We all have dreams—big dreams of what we want out of life, smaller dreams of relationships we wish to develop, skills we wish to master, self-understanding we wish to cultivate, adventures we want to pursue, and changes we want to make. Goals carry us from dreaming to doing by giving us purpose and direction. They also provide a rationale and a set of priorities to guide us in selecting which changes we want to make when.

As road maps that lead to dreams, goals provide a destination and, at the least, suggest an itinerary for getting there. Once you decide that you want to make a personal change in your life, setting goals is the best way of getting from Point A to Point B—and eventually all the way to Point Z.

Without goals, you remain what you were. With goals, you become what you wish. This chapter presents the most effective strategies for crafting and using goals to map your way to the life you want.

Your Big Picture

Big ideas and big dreams energize and motivate us by making the work of change worthwhile. Only when we allow and encourage big-picture thinking in ourselves do we begin to stretch and extend beyond what we consider our limits. By directing all of your potential toward something that gets your juices flowing, goals provide a focal point for your efforts. A dream or a compelling big-picture vision helps you engage fully and melts away irritations, obstacles, and inconveniences.

Give yourself this advantage. Begin to think in terms of dreams and constructing a life that is the stuff of dreams. This won't just happen. You have to make it happen through your choices and your actions. Choices create the specific blueprint for converting your big picture from a blue-sky fantasy to the bedrock upon which you build. By having a dream, you will know which changes to make and which actions to take. Make the changes you need to reach your big-picture dream of the life you want.

Be Specific

Ending world hunger and saving the environment are worthy dreams, but how do you work toward such hazy ideals? You don't—unless and until you convert them into steps you can complete. You need to state your guiding dreams in language that is believable, precise, and tangible enough that you can convert them into goals, subgoals, and action steps.

JOURNALING ASSIGNMENT : Dream Big

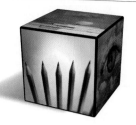

If you already know your dream, write it in your *Journal for An Invitation to Personal Change*.

If you do not have a specific dream or vision yet, the following exercise will help you create one. As quickly as you can, write down in your *IPC Journal* your vision, your big-picture dream, and your wildest, most outrageous, even your most far-fetched hopes and goals. (Yes, you can include becoming a rock star, a professional athlete, a CEO, or the President.) Do not judge or edit—just keep writing until you have written everything you can think of.

_____

_____

_____

_____

_____

_____

Now write answers to the following questions. Write quickly, allowing no more than 60 to 90 seconds for every answer. If an answer doesn't come to you in that time, skip the question and move on to the next one.

1. What do you want your life to be like?

_____

_____

_____

_____

_____

_____

2. What draws your attention and taps into your enthusiasm? What fascinates you, intrigues you, or tickles your curiosity?

_____

_____

_____

_____

_____

_____

3. What would you do if you were guaranteed 100 percent success?

_____

_____

_____

_____

_____

_____

4. If you had the self-esteem necessary to be unstoppable, what would you do differently?

_____

_____

_____

_____

_____

_____

5. As a child, what did you first seriously imagine you would do when you grew up? What was your first true ambition?

_____

_____

_____

_____

_____

_____

6. What qualities continue to inspire respect and awe in you? What qualities would you develop in yourself if you knew how?

_____

_____

_____

_____

_____

_____

7. What would you plan to do in the future if you didn't have to earn money to make a living?

_____

_____

_____

_____

_____

_____

Look at these questions daily and keep answering them until you hit pay dirt or run out of new things to say. If you can answer all of them the first day, fine. If you draw a blank on one or more of them, take another look the next day and see what comes to you. Don't worry about not answering right away. Whether the questions remain consciously on your mind or not, trust us: they continue to work outside your conscious awareness.

If after a week you can't come up with one specific dream, write a list of the things you want to do, experience, or master before you die. Choose one idea from this list to use as your vision as you continue working through this chapter.

VISUALIZATION : See Your Dream

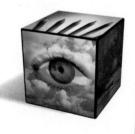

The brain, as neuroscientists have discovered, does not distinguish between what you visualize and what you actually see. Imagining something, such as a friend's face, activates the same areas of the brain in the same way as actually seeing the person. If seeing is believing, so is visualizing. Take advantage of this neural quirk by visualizing good outcomes rather than negative ones and seeing yourself completing the actions necessary to create them. Do the following exercise daily. (There is no endpoint. You can keep doing it for the rest of your life.)

Visualize in detail as often as possible specific scenes that depict what your life will be like when you are living your dream. For example, if you want to become the next Steve Jobs, you could imagine yourself dazzling an audience with a breakthrough gadget so innovative it makes the iPhone look as old-fashioned as a hand-cranked record player.

The more vividly you can see, feel, touch, and taste your dream, the more likely you are to achieve it. Relax. For a few minutes, allow yourself inside the world you are aiming to enter. See your surroundings, the furnishings, or the landscape; notice smells, the quality of the air, and the way you feel in your body. Notice what you are wearing in your dream world and how your clothing feels as it caresses your skin.

Then view yourself doing things that relate to and express your dream. Pay attention to how this makes you feel. Notice the time of day. Hear the sounds. See yourself from the outside, as if you are watching a movie, and from the inside, as if you have entered the movie and are watching it unfold before your eyes. Enjoy the sensations and affirm to yourself that this is your life. When you have finished the visualization, stretch, open your eyes, and return to the physical world.

As you use this powerful tool in the chapters that follow, remember to involve senses besides vision. Additional details make the experience more vivid. If for some reason you are not satisfied with a particular visualization, don't fret. You will become more adept and at ease with visualizations as you use them.

▶ ### Ask the Big-Picture Questions

Once you've identified your big vision or dream, ask yourself two simple but powerful questions every day:

1. What did I do today to fulfill my vision?

    _____

    _____

    _____

    _____

    _____

    _____

2. When the answer is "nothing," ask yourself, what did I make more important than my vision, and why?

    _____

    _____

    _____

    _____

    _____

    _____

These two questions can help you stay on target to reach any goal.

_____

Your Master Plan for Getting to Your Goals and Dreams

Thinking and talking won't get you to your goals; planning and doing will. Whether you want to become a triathlete or start a moving business with your friends, your master plan must include each of the following steps. Do them now.

1. Break down your ultimate goal into projects.

_____

_____

_____

_____

_____

_____

_____

_____

2. Break down each project into tasks.

_____

_____

_____

_____

_____

_____

_____

_____

_____

_____

3. Break down tasks into manageable action steps.

_____

_____

_____

_____

_____

_____

_____

_____

_____

_____

_____

4. Start with simple action steps and progress to more advanced ones. Think of yourself as climbing a staircase, one step at a time.

_____

_____

_____

_____

_____

_____

_____

_____

5. Break down each action step into specific activities that can be completed in discrete, manageable chunks of time.

_____

_____

_____

_____

_____

_____

_____

_____

By taking these actions, you will easily generate a master plan that converts even fuzzy wishes into specific actions. Fill out the plan with all other essential details you will need to make it complete and workable.

Your master plan can take whatever form you wish. Depending on your objective, your master plan could be as spare and simple as a one- or two-page list, a flowchart, or a project board. Or it could be more complex. Be creative. People vary widely in how much structure they want or feel they need. You may find that you benefit from far more detailed preparation and structure than you have used in the past. If your goal requires many separate steps, simply spelling them all out will require detail.

The master plan exists to serve you, not shackle you. It is a tool for reaching a goal but is not the goal itself. To be helpful, your master plan needs to go beyond providing merely general guidelines and directions. The objective is to create a succinct, step-by-step recipe that leaves nothing out and ensures that your efforts are pragmatic and efficient.

Make your master plan systematic and thorough enough that it eliminates "seat of the pants" approximations and guesstimates. Remember the carpenter's maxim: "Measure twice, cut once."

The following questions can help you prepare. Answer them in your *IPC Journal* or in the space below:

1. What skills do I need to achieve this?

_____

_____

_____

_____

_____

_____

_____

_____

_____

_____

_____

2. What information and knowledge must I acquire?

_____

_____

_____

_____

_____

_____

_____

_____

_____

_____

3. What help, assistance, or resources do I need?

_____

_____

_____

_____

_____

_____

_____

_____

4. What could block my progress? (For each potential barrier, list solutions.)

_____

_____

_____

_____

_____

_____

_____

_____

5. Who or what could I allow to get in my way? (For each potential barrier, list solutions.)

_____

_____

_____

_____

_____

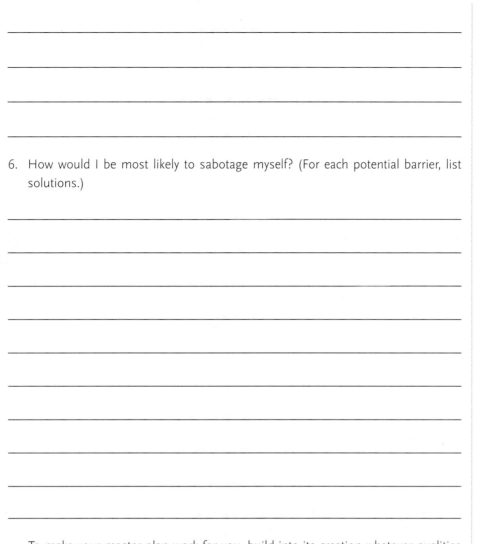

_____

_____

_____

_____

6. How would I be most likely to sabotage myself? (For each potential barrier, list solutions.)

_____

_____

_____

_____

_____

_____

_____

_____

_____

To make your master plan work for you, build into its creation whatever qualities will ensure success. If you've skipped steps and taken shortcuts in the past, go for broke on precision and detail. If, on the other hand, you have gotten stuck at the planning stage, correct that by cutting to the chase. Busywork can be as big an evasion as any other form of postponing. Do not turn planning and preparation into a way of becoming terminally stuck. Develop a straightforward plan, and then get started. You can always make adjustments as you go along.

You can organize a master plan by envisioning what you want to do, the steps involved in achieving it, and the probable difficulties. Or you can do it the other way around by imagining the final destination and working backward. In either case, write down every step.

Make the final version of your master plan attractive. If you started by making notes on paper napkins, fine. Many creative projects begin this way. But transfer your plan to some good-quality, durable medium, such as your _IPC Journal,_ and make it neat and clean. Pay it a certain respect.

When you plan with attention to detail, you exercise your capacity to think realistically and concretely about time, and you develop your ability to think about and simplify the process of reaching seemingly unreachable goals. Over time this kind of thinking leads to the development of quiet confidence.

As you develop your master plan, make sure each goal is within your control. Other people should not have to change in order for you to meet your goal. Don't expect your roommate to jump on your end-global-warming bandwagon or your best friend to sizzle with the same enthusiasm for volunteering at a local soup kitchen. If your company is paying your tuition, you can't assume your boss will rubber-stamp your plan to take a term off for travel.

Focus on the process, not the outcome. If you sign up for a weekend tai chi seminar because your health teacher is the instructor, set the goal of acquiring the new skill set (something you can control) rather than impressing your instructor (something you cannot).

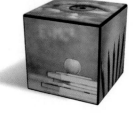

CLASSROOM ACTIVITY : Share Your Master Plan

Objective feedback can play an invaluable role in helping you reach the short-term goals that lead you to your long-term goals. Work with a partner in your class, and take a hard look at each other's master plan. Is each plan clear enough to follow easily? Can you eliminate gaps, fuzziness, and loopholes? Trim unnecessary steps? Insert missing ones? Rather than investing days in revising and rewriting your plan on your own, let your partner evaluate what additional work it may need.

Become a Goal-Getter

People who set goals, write them down, and review them reach them faster. They also report that they are happier and gain more satisfaction from life. Learn when and how to set goals, and you will move toward your goals more quickly.

Goals come in two forms: long-range or destination goals and short-range goals. Your long-range goals provide the overall perspective that shapes all other aspects of your decision making. You wouldn't board a bus without knowing where you want to go, but it's easy to drift along in life with only a vague sense of where you're heading.

Owning Your Goals

Whenever you're setting goals—whether long term or short term—two guidelines are critical:

▌ Set only your own goals. Don't allow others to set them for you, and don't set goals for others.
▌ Always write your goals down, and look at them often. Putting a goal in writing moves you from wishing to doing, from contemplation to preparation and action. When you write goals down, you become more committed to making your words come true.

JOURNALING ASSIGNMENT : Setting Long-Term Goals

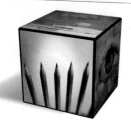

A long-term goal transforms your brain into a satellite dish picking up the signals that are most relevant to your quest. Rather than staying in the "wouldn't it be nice if...." mode, a destination goal instructs your mind to focus on an objective. Then, while you get to work on the short-term goals and action steps, your unconscious mind searches for additional possibilities and creative solutions.

For reasons we discuss more fully later, we suggest keeping your big-picture dream or vision private and allowing others to do the same. For now, simply realize that dreams, because of their distant and imaginative scope, can be squelched by the dismissive or disbelieving comments of others. This is especially true when the vision is ambitious, newly formed, or still in the process of being fleshed out.

1. Review your descriptions of your dreams and visions, and translate them into one overarching dream and a handful of specific, long-term goals. If your dream were a career in Chinese studies, one obvious long-term goal would be to become fluent in Mandarin.

2. Turn your vision into a goal by writing, "I am fluent in Mandarin." Setting goals in the right way increases their effectiveness, so write your long-term goals in the present tense as if you've already achieved them. In doing this, you put your mind to work to make your desired change happen in the present. Don't fret about whether you're lying to yourself.

   As we explain in greater depth in Chapter 7, the way we use language affects the brain's responses. For example, if you say, "I have blue eyes," you presume that you will continue to have blue eyes into the future. Likewise, if you say, "I am a Chinese scholar," the present tense instructs the unconscious mind on what to bring about and then sustain.

3. Write no more than five or six long-term goals in this fashion.

4. Do not set a time limit for these goals. The reason? If you set a deadline for a long-term goal, you may slow your progress by eliminating opportunities for your unconscious mind to find truly creative and efficient solutions that could come more quickly. You don't want to direct your mind to wait until some stated time if it can come up with results sooner.

5. To ensure that your unconscious mind pays attention to your goals, repeat each goal five times in the morning and five times at night until you reach it. This exercise makes your long-term goal function as a command directing you to make efforts toward meeting it.

Setting Short-Term Goals

Short-term goals are tools for reaching immediate objectives in brief time frames, such as one week. An example of short-term goal planning might be to make six phone calls, check certain websites, or read a certain book within a week.

A short-term goal has specific objectives and an unambiguous deadline for meeting it. It differs from a long-term goal in one additional way: You deliberately make it public. As you'll see in Chapter 11, we suggest telling someone who agrees to hold you accountable to achieving your goal by the deadline you set.

Here are some additional guidelines:

1. Decide on specific objectives you want to accomplish within a brief period, such as one week, and write them down. For instance, you may want to discover and evaluate all Chinese-language groups or activities on campus.
2. Schedule time to accomplish your goal. You might set aside time between classes to meet with a Chinese language professor.
3. Announce your goals to one other person. Agree to check in with him or her at a specific time every week to report on your progress and to set new goals to reach by your next meeting.
4. Schedule time to look at your list of short-term goals every day, and take the actions necessary to reach them. Make this a nonnegotiable imperative.
5. Whenever you achieve a goal, check it off, tell a friend, or just raise your hands above your head like an athlete who's just clinched a championship. This builds your sense of "I can do it. I am doing it. Look how far I've come!"

▶ *Don't Settle for Halfway*

Despite good intentions and considerable progress, many people give up their goals just before the rainbow's end—and congratulate themselves for getting that far. Would you ever board a plane for Chicago and say, "Well, we got three-quarters of the way there!" as if that were good? Persist, persevere, and don't settle for almost there. If you stall on the final stretch, do a quick reality check. Maybe you need to add some smaller step goals, seek more support, or simply allow yourself more time.

Real Change: Second Time Around (continued)

When Nate, whom you met on page 12 of Chapter 1, went back to college, his big dream was a better life for himself and his family. But he soon realized he needed specific goals to convert his dream into a blueprint. As Nate began the exercises in this chapter, one question brought him to a dead halt: "What would you do if you were guaranteed 100 percent success?" He thought back to the jobs that had given him the most satisfaction. Almost all involved "green" construction projects that used cutting-edge technology to reduce carbon emissions and take advantage of energy-saving design. Ever since becoming a father, Nate had been thinking about the world his children would inherit. What if he could do something to leave the planet in better shape?

Nate's big-picture dream became a set of specific goals when he decided to prepare for a career in ecological engineering. Knowing what he wanted and how to get there galvanized Nate. He developed a master plan, starting with the project of getting into a state university with a good department in ecological engineering and a series of subprojects, such as completing his general education requirements at his community college. He further broke down this project into manageable action steps, such as calculating how many credits he could reasonably carry in a term. He developed a list of skills he should acquire, information and knowledge he could use, and assistance or resources he would need.

When he looks back to his first round at college, Nate realizes that he had no direction and no dream. Now that he is clear about what he wants, he no longer fears that he is too old to go back to school or that he can't handle the academic challenge. In fact, school is turning out to be easier than he thought because he is focused. Nate now sees himself as standing at the foot of a staircase. One step at a time, he is sure he will get to the top.

Power Journaling

These days everyone seems to have something to say—and is putting it out there in blogs, vlogs, MySpace, wiki pages, YouTube, you name it. More than 8 in 10 college students have a profile on Facebook; most log in at least once a week. With so much sharing of likes, dislikes, thoughts, wishes, and much too much information, what's left to say?

Plenty—especially when you're writing to and for only you. *Journaling*—the process of putting feelings and thoughts into written words—is an industrial strength power tool for behavior change. This form of expressive writing provides an opportunity to reflect; evaluate past, present, and future behavior; and gain insight into your feelings. As more than a decade of research has shown, writing about your inner life also has a positive effect on both mental and physical health.

We will help you make journaling the secret weapon in your personal change program through exercises that appear in each chapter. Your *Journal for An Invitation to Personal Change* is designed as a "starter" journal to get you going. But we suggest that you continue to journal long after you finish this class and get your degree. (Why ever stop?) This chapter helps you overcome any resistance to this type of writing, offers simple how-to steps, and suggests an array of ways to journal. At least one is certain to appeal to you, but we suggest that you give each of them a try.

Overcoming Journalphobia

Some people scorn journaling because it isn't action oriented enough. Maybe you think having a diary is something kids do in fifth grade. Maybe you can't imagine what you could gain from writing about your thoughts and experiences. Think again.

Certain individuals—men more than women—resist personal writing until some traumatic experience, such as a breakup, serious illness, or the death of a friend or loved one, forces them to seek deeper understanding. But don't wait for a crisis. Even everyday frustrations and victories can provide topics for your writing. Journaling works every time you use it—not just in emergencies.

Have you ever tried but failed to communicate the excitement of a truly extraordinary experience? Maybe the best you could manage was, "You had to be there." Journaling is another "had to be there" phenomenon. You have to do it to understand it. Simply keeping track of your experiences and observations can lead to a profound inner exploration—and to personal change.

Your journal is personal, not for public display. Make sure that the people you live with—family members or roommates—know that your journal is your private property. You will find that others will be respectful of your writing, especially when you ask them to treat it that way.

Five Steps to Get Going

1. If you have your *IPC Journal,* great. If not, use the space that follows, and start writing.
2. Continue for at least 15 minutes.
3. Don't worry about spelling or grammar or how much or how little you write.
4. Remember that your words are for your eyes only. Don't censor yourself.
5. For this entry, just pour out everything that comes to mind about journaling—whether you've ever done it, why you think you'll like it or hate it, and so on. Let it all hang out.

_____

_____

_____

_____

_____

_____

_____

_____

_____

_____

_____

_____

_____

_____

_____

_____

_____

_____

_____

_____

_____

_____

Whether you are saying to yourself that this exercise was good, bad, or in between, it really was a start (unless you already journal). So don't stop here. Keep it up. In about three weeks (at most) you will begin to observe changes that may surprise you.

Journaling as a Force

Some people use journaling from time to time to tap into creativity and solve specific problems. Nothing wrong with that. But we are suggesting journaling as an ongoing tool for personal change and greater self-understanding.

This type of journaling can truly empower you. Why? Here is what we know:

- People are on the run but seldom know the big picture of where they are going. Journaling provides the opportunity to step back. It's another way of getting to know yourself and of acquiring a bird's-eye view on where you are now and where you want to go from here. Journaling serves as an ongoing GPS-type tool that can keep you on course.

- We are drowning in information. Facts of every conceivable type are at our fingertips. Want to know the temperature in Prague? You know how to get it. Just Google. Want to settle a bet on which league won the most World Series titles in the last 20 years? All it takes is a couple of keystrokes. Yet we are profoundly short of self-knowledge. Journaling, if you stay with it, taps into deeper understanding and wisdom and takes you beyond just emotional intelligence to weave a tapestry of personal reflections that inform all your decisions and judgments.

- Without reflection and contemplation, we are highly likely to repeat what we have always done. We are far more susceptible to following instead of leading and to acting on impulse or habit instead of reason. Journaling creates an opportunity to reflect. And reflection is a crucial part of a four-step process of gathering information before making a decision:

  1. Think.
  2. Ask someone's advice and consent.
  3. Think again and reflect.
  4. Decide.

- Journaling is an antidote to media saturation, gimmickry, and blind materialism. Commercials screech at you; news teasers bait you; the Internet beckons you. But none leads to depth or understanding. There is more to life than news, weather, sports, celebrity gossip, and reality shows. You already know this, but journaling is a power tool for getting to what else exists. Deeper satisfactions arise from self-knowledge than from any TV show or video game.

- Journaling, when practiced regularly, taps your unconscious and your creativity in ways that are surprising and not immediately clear. Do you have to understand electricity to flip a switch and turn on lights? No. Nor do you have to understand why journaling can improve your grades, your relationships, or your coping skills. But it may do all of this and more.

Jump-Start Your Journaling

If you don't know where to start, it doesn't matter. You could start journaling about football or TV cooking shows. If you kept tracking your feelings about them, it would eventually take you to core beliefs you might never have otherwise discovered. To jump-start your journaling, complete one of the following sentences in your *IPC Journal:*

1. When I think about my life, I wish I had _____

   _____

   _____

   _____

   _____

   _____

2. When I reflect on my habits, they seem _____

   _____

   _____

   _____

   _____

   _____

3. Thinking about the way I handle relationships, I feel _____

   _____

   _____

   _____

   _____

   _____

   _____

Maximum Impact Journaling

No, you don't need to put pen to paper. You can create a new computer file. Or you can talk into a tape recorder. However, seeing words in print carries a more powerful subconscious impact. Whatever the method, as long as you put your thoughts and feelings into words on a regular basis, you will benefit. But for maximum benefit, if you can afford it, we recommend the following:

1. *Use your IPC Journal as your "starter" journal.* Don't try to get by with a yellow legal pad. Your *IPC Journal* provides high-quality paper and a design created to appeal and beckon to you.
2. *Get an excellent writing instrument.* Find something that feels good in your hand and looks good to your eye. An elegant writing instrument is to journaling as silver flatware is to a good meal. You can eat good food from a plastic fork, but it takes

the experience down several notches. Do everything to make journaling an occasion, like a fine meal.

3. *Write at a particular time of day and for a period you specify in advance.* Journaling at a fixed time of day strengthens the habit and becomes a pleasant date with yourself to anticipate. Journaling for a fixed period forces you to go deeper. It means that you do not quit at the first distraction. We strongly recommend that you write first thing in the morning or last thing at night—or better yet, both.

    If you write first thing in the morning, you tap directly into your mind when it is fresh, rested, and free of the distractions and mechanical habits of the day. If you write at night, you have a chance to survey the day and process what happened. While you sleep, the mind can assimilate and work without interference on the material you just provided.

4. *Write regularly.* More is better than less. Daily is better than occasionally. You don't have to write every day, although we do suggest a minimum of four or five times a week. On the other hand, would you brush your teeth only four or five days a week? Think of journaling as brushing your mind.

Journal Topics

Selecting a topic for a journal provides a focal point. You will find that if you write about one subject day after day, you will penetrate that topic to an unprecedented degree. As you write about a topic long enough, you will write about the way it relates to your life, your career, and your goals.

We recommend that you try journaling on one topic for a while before shifting, but do eventually move to different topics and aspects of your life. For example, if you do not understand your emotional reactions, keep a running record of intense feelings you have in the course of the day. Do not immediately look for patterns. As you write over time, they will clearly emerge and you will begin to see what you have been allowing to set you off. Then you can intelligently plan how to deal with your reactions.

Here are some other ideas:

- Your relationships
- Films
- Books
- Dreams
- Your job
- Curiosities
- Emotions (negative and positive)
- Goals
- Ways you might serve a cause or community

Add a few ideas of your own:

- _____
- _____
- _____
- _____

Stumped? The following assignment can get your started.

JOURNALING ASSIGNMENT : Journaling for Better Health and Wellness

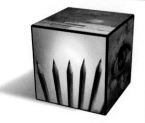

Once you've identified a target health goal, write it in your journal. Then do the following exercise:

1. Identify your best health habits. Write down everything you are doing to improve your health and wellness.

_____

_____

_____

_____

_____

_____

_____

_____

_____

_____

2. Honestly list your worst health habits. Write down what you are doing that is not good for your body, mind, or spirit.

_____

_____

_____

_____

_____

_____

_____

_____

_____

_____

3. Ask yourself and answer in writing: What is one thing you could do to improve your health and enhance your wellness?

_____

_____

_____

4. What could you do right away?

_____

_____

_____

5. Today?

_____

_____

_____

6. This week?

_____

_____

_____

7. This month?

_____

_____

_____

8. Write down one thing that you will do, as soon as possible, to improve your health.

_____

_____

_____

CLASS ACTIVITY : Group Journaling

With your classmates, create a blog or wiki page in which to journal about journaling and about the other tools you will learn to use during your personal change experiences.

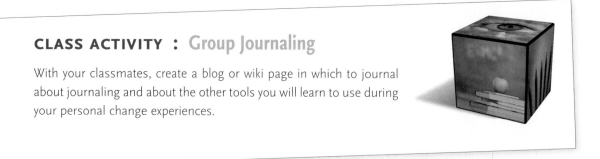

Types of Journaling

We encourage you to experiment with various types of writing in your journal. Here are some ideas for you to try.

Stream-of-Consciousness Journaling

In stream-of-consciousness journaling, you simply record whatever thoughts come into your mind. Sit quietly and breathe deeply. Once relaxed and settled, begin to write. Don't be surprised at the number and intensity of thoughts and feelings that emerge. As they become part of your awareness, they may lead to insights that have eluded you in the past because you are not taking the time to "hear" what you are thinking.

Journaling for Specific Solutions

You also can use your journal to tackle specific issues and challenges.

- Write when you need to sort out complicated feelings about an issue in your life.
- Write when you're struggling to persist with a change.
- Write before an activity that may challenge your commitment to change, for instance, before joining your friends on a Friday night after you've committed yourself to not smoking or overeating.
- Write afterward or the next day to chronicle the good choices you made or to note what you'll do differently the next time.

Reflective Journaling

Try reflective journaling and write about yourself and your life in the third person. You might begin with the phrase, "It was a time when…." Describe an event or experience in detail, using as many of your senses as possible. Write down the sounds, sights, smells, and feelings as if you were writing a novel. Use "he" or "she," rather than "I," as if you were an outside observer. Often this provides a new perspective on what you're going through.

Cathartic Writing

Let it all out. Put your pain, fear, anger, frustrations, and grief down on paper. Say what you want or need to say on the page. The journal is a safe place where no one will judge or criticize you. Begin with the phrase, "Right now I feel….," then let yourself write whatever comes out. If you run out of feelings, reread what you've just written and then write the next thing that comes to mind.

After you release deep emotions, you may choose to throw away your writing or burn it as a rite of letting go of an event or feeling that disrupted your life. Follow your intuition's lead as to what to do with the words once you've written them.

You don't have to wait until you're feeling bad to write. Use your journal to celebrate feelings of joy and gratitude. (As we discuss in "The Grateful Thread" lab in the *Labs for An Invitation to Personal Change,* keeping a gratitude journal is one of the best ways of boosting your mood.)

Letters You Never Send

Write a letter in your journal to a person, place, event, even an attitude. By allowing you to express emotions that you may not feel comfortable venting more directly, this technique can allow you to resolve issues with someone who is far away or dead or to process difficult emotions, such as anger or frustration, that come up in a relationship.

Begin with a salutation, just as you would if you were writing a letter: "Dear...." Then let your pen lead you. You may be surprised at the power and clarity you experience from your writing. While you are writing or afterward, you may feel deep emotions. Accept them as normal and healthy. In fact, the emotional release contributes to the healthy impact of journaling. If you want to do more with what you've written, share it with a trusted friend or counselor.

Dialogue Journaling

You might experiment with dialogue journaling, in which you split yourself into two or more identities. In essence, you compose a script with at least two characters. One character might talk only of the benefits of making a personal change. The other might complain about the drawbacks and difficulties. A third might comment on the exchange between the other two. Write a back-and-forth conversation, giving each character equal opportunity to make points and counterpoints.

Resist Your Resistance

If you're resisting the idea of journaling, you are putting off its many benefits. Here is what to do. Write a journal entry now. If you do not have your *IPC Journal* with you, use the space that follows. Keep going. Do not stop.

You may take to journaling unbelievably quickly despite your doubts. On the other hand, if you get distracted and the whole thing mostly seems silly, push past that. Trust us on this. The experiences that you resist the most are usually among the most powerful tools you wind up using. Do not quit. Keep auditioning types of journaling until you get the one perfect for the part. It's just a matter of time and casting.

_____

_____

_____

_____

_____

_____

_____

_____

_____

_____

_____

_____

_____

_____

_____

_____

_____

_____

_____

_____

_____

Journal Writing Links

If you want to explore journaling further and find out how others use it for personal growth, check out some of the following Internet sites. If any of the following links are no longer valid, you should be able to find similar ones with a little research:

Inspired to Journal
http://www.kporterfield.com/journal/Journal_Links.html

Living: A Monthly Oasis of Healing and Joy
http://www.s oulfulliving.com/

Conversations Within: Journal Writing and Inner Dialog
http://www.gerrystarnes.com/journal/

Journal for You
http://www.journalforyou.com/

Diarist.net
http://www.diarist.net/

Journal Writers
http://www.rightmindlogic.com/index.htm

Writing the Journey
http://www.writingthejourney.com/

Open Directory List of Journal Links
http://dmoz.org/Arts/Online_Writing/Journals/Resources

Real change: test terror (continued)

At first Malika, whom you read about on page 26 of Chapter 2, didn't see the point of talking to herself, which is what she thought of writing in a journal. But one evening after the girls were asleep, she picked up a pen and wrote, "What scares me most about tests is.... not knowing the answers." So what do you do when you don't know the answers? The teaching assistant's curt advice echoed in Malika's brain: You study.

Malika turned to the "Defusing Test Stress" lab in her copy of the *IPC Labs*. By working through the exercises, she changed her approach to studying so that she could convert what she learned into practical knowledge. As she continued to journal, Malika realized that she had accepted her mother's description of her as a poor test taker as the truth without bothering to find out what skills she needed to perform better on exams. Most importantly, she came to see that she had developed an automatic panicky reaction to the first sign of difficulty, which blocked her thoughts and information she knew.

The morning of her next midterm, Malika practiced deep-breathing exercises on the way to campus. As soon as she read the first question, she felt herself relax: She knew the answer. She struggled a bit on the second question. As her heart started to pound, she told herself to come back to it later. After completing two questions with some mastery, Malika returned to the one she'd skipped and noticed that she had made it more difficult than it was. She focused on demonstrating what she did know rather than panicking because she couldn't remember a specific fact or two.

The result? Malika got an 89—and felt a strong sense of satisfaction. It was the beginning of a new feeling of confidence based on her realization that test taking is a skill to learn and improve, not an inherent ability you either have or don't.

CHAPTER 10

Making Yourself Lucky

Go ahead and buy the lottery ticket. Bet on the big game. Wish on a shooting star. You might get lucky. Or you can read your horoscope, throw the *I Ching* for clues to the future, or simply wait and watch your fate unfold. Just don't count on these approaches bringing you what you want in life.

As we discussed in Chapter 2, people with an internal locus or sense of control act as if life is a game of skill rather than chance. They go through life assuming that they are the director and, to the greatest extent possible, take charge of the movie that is their life. They do not see themselves as omnipotent. They know that other factors play into life, but they never miss any chance to exercise control. Those with an external locus of control, on the other hand, are passive. They see themselves as movie extras, bit players, mere spectators swept along by luck or fate.

As hundreds of studies have shown, you're better off in the director's chair. "Internals" act more independently, enjoy better health, are more optimistic—and are more successful at personal change. Regardless of how lucky or unlucky you think you may be, this chapter teaches you how to make your own luck by making the most of every opportunity that presents itself and seeing opportunity where others fail to see it.

Build Your Personal Power to Change

Remember the story of Robinson Crusoe? Shipwrecked on a desert island, he had to change in order to survive. His original destination and goals no longer mattered. He had to deal with a new reality. He did so by using the island and the boat wreckage to provide everything he needed to survive. Instead of mourning what he lost, he played the hand he was dealt to its maximum advantage. If he had done otherwise and spent his time grieving for what should or might have been, he would have perished.

When you're facing a challenge or a change (or the challenge of change), think like Robinson Crusoe: Use what you've got. Take advantage of every opportunity. Don't snivel. Don't pine for something you lack, like more money or a supportive partner. Become the master of what you have and what is available to you.

Exploit the advantages of what seem to be disadvantages. If you feel that you don't have enough money, for example, become expert at stretching your resources. Use your student ID to get into museums and movies at a lower price. Investigate all the free classes, craft studios, movies, music and dance facilities, recreational programs, and other opportunities available on campus. Go to art fairs on the quad. Enjoy free concerts by student choruses and bands. Buy vintage rather than new. If you have children, play ball, dominoes, and checkers with them rather than shelling out major money for PlayStation. You don't need an extravagant budget. Pay attention and you will be awash in great opportunities for special experiences. Remember: Every sunset is free, and there's no charge for walking in the moonlight.

If you're thinking ahead to your career (and you should be), you may worry about how to go about getting job experience. Rather than hustling for whatever low-paying job you can scrounge, volunteer to work for free doing something you find meaningful or with someone you admire. Once you get that opportunity, become as useful and productive as you can. Do not fall victim to conventional thinking—your own or someone else's—about what you must achieve on what timetable.

Act on what you *have* now and where you *are* now. You may become so valuable to the organization for which you volunteer that when you say you can't afford to stay longer they offer you a paying job because they don't want to lose you. Whether they do or not, you will have had an experience and a chance to learn in the environment you were seeking.

Do everything you can with whatever is at your disposal and exploit every opportunity to achieve your goals. Think like an Olympian: Although most Olympic athletes are born with natural talent, all must work hard to develop their agility, strength, skills, and mental toughness. The best, the strongest, the swiftest, and the most skilled would never make it to the Olympics, let alone to the medal stand, if they did not make the most of what they have.

This book is designed to move you toward greater personal power. The rest of this chapter provides specific methods that build your power to exert control and thereby increase your personal efficacy.

Shape Up for Change

If you want to build cardiorespiratory or aerobic fitness, you could take up running. If you decide to do so, it's best to start by going a short distance at a slow speed. If you push yourself to go too far too fast, you're likely to injure yourself or quit. The same is true with any personal change.

To build your emotional stamina for the long haul, start small. Each day find one thing that you began at some point but have not yet finished. Your assignment? Simply complete this "incomplete."

Your chore does not have to be something big and might take less than five minutes—folding the towels you washed last weekend, returning the DVDs you borrowed from a friend, paying your cell phone bill online. Most college students have such a stash of incompletes that they can do this exercise for a long time without running out of tasks. If you also work or have children, you may have a lifetime supply.

As you proceed, observe the surprising immediate effects. You probably feel an unexpected boost. The reason? Incompletes suck energy. Completing them releases the energy they monopolize. You will feel lighter and more energetic from the first completion the very first day.

When you have done this exercise daily for three weeks, add the following exercise: Begin one mildly unpleasant thing that stretches you a bit. Do not attempt too big a step. And select something only slightly difficult.

Don't groan. Don't protest. Stay with us. We will not ask you to crawl over cut glass or endure pointless physical challenges like a reality show contestant. But we do want you to experience what happens when you take on a mild dose of challenge instead of postponing or evading it.

To complete this exercise, you could choose to do something practical that you find unpleasant, such as alphabetizing your CDs or organizing your underwear and sock drawers, or something impractical and pointless, such as packing paper clips neatly in a small box and then unpacking them.

But why not kill two birds with the same stone? Why not do something practical that will simultaneously further your academic success? For instance, study for the class you find most difficult as early as possible in the day. In addition to completing one incomplete every day, faithfully add this mild stretch activity to your daily routine for three weeks and observe the effects.

Note that choosing to do first what you might otherwise have done last creates immediate payoffs. For starters, you complete the more challenging study task when you are freshest. This alone can create a positive ripple effect. Handling tough course material early can make it easier to comprehend. When you understand the content better, you may enjoy the work and the class more. As a bonus, your grade may improve as well.

Second, you send yourself powerful positive messages about your ability to handle something difficult. Talk about getting bang for your buck! This kind of impact for the effort expended is what we mean by a power tool.

As you work on these tasks, the work you do works on you. By practicing simple exercises repetitively, you increase your tenacity and persistence and, in the process, make your locus of control more internal. You will be well on your way to mastering the tool of making your own luck.

See the Steps of Change

If you imagine a hypothetical event, such as winning an award or being selected to manage a project, you are more likely to consider it possible and make it happen. In studies of world-class athletes, those who practiced positive visualization performed better than those who exercised just as much but did not use this psychological technique.

However, it's important to visualize not just the final moment of triumph but also the actual steps and activities that lead up to it. As social psychology research has shown, if you visualize yourself completing the various steps of a project just before sitting down to it, you will be more likely to complete your work in the allotted time.

Olympic gold-medal hurdler Edwin Moses used to visualize an entire 400-meter hurdle race, imagining every single stride he would take, seeing himself crossing each hurdle, and then envisioning himself sprinting to the finish line. Sports psychologists contend that his visualization of the entire race was more effective than just imagining the moment when the gold medal slipped over his head. Visualizing the steps of any process creates a readiness to complete the process just as you've imagined it.

If your goal is to get to a healthier weight, visualize yourself waking up full of confidence and determination. See yourself selecting and enjoying making a meal of healthier, less-processed foods. See yourself eating slowly, enjoying each bite, and pushing back your plate when you first start to feel full. Visualize yourself sipping from a water bottle throughout the day. See yourself changing into workout clothes and jogging along your favorite path or putting in time in the weight room. Notice the sensations within your body and the sights and sounds around you.

Practice your positive visualization at least twice a day, once in the morning and once in the evening. The more detailed your vision of your positive behaviors, the more benefits you'll derive from the exercise. End each visualization with your personal equivalent of an Olympic gold medal—whether that's stepping on the scale with a smile, crossing the finish line of a charity fun run, or acing a test.

▶ See Yourself

Before you begin any task, visualize briefly how you want to conduct yourself during the activity. Let's say it's time to study for that tough literature test. Before you begin studying, visualize yourself taking notes or underlining passages. See yourself writing practice essays with interest, enthusiasm, and comprehension. Inject a mild note of urgency; add a great deal of attention. Then just do it.

Intensify Your Attention

The college experience offers endless enticements and distractions, from the hottie in your spin class to the campus anime film festival. Every day you could find ingenious and mundane ways to pass and to waste time. This alone is one reason to cultivate your ability to focus your attention.

The more you learn to stay on task, the more efficient you become at everything from homework to housework. You don't want to spend your time at the library reading then rereading the same page from intro psych for 20 minutes. If you finish your work in an intensive fashion, you will have more guilt-free time for flirting or yoga.

Mindfulness, a term used to describe any method that involves paying attention to what you are doing and experiencing, improves the quality of everything you do, large or small. Washing a single window pane with exquisite attention is refreshing because the mind craves use in the same way that muscles crave activity. Intensifying attention, helpful in all types of circumstances, makes you luckier by providing access to information you need to direct change.

Becoming more aware of what is happening within and around you accelerates the transition from the precontemplation stage to the contemplation stage of change. By observing subtle feelings and sensations, you recognize what is bubbling up in the background of your consciousness. When you understand the nature of your discontent or yearning, you have more personal power to make and direct steps toward change. By tuning in to your inner world and paying close attention to the external world, you see possibilities to exploit and ways to complete assignments and other tasks more efficiently. When you perceive more clearly what you prefer, you can better create experiences that satisfy you.

When you are not actively engaging in a mindfulness exercise, such as those described in the "Rx: Relax" and "Mind over Platter" labs, make it a practice to infuse all your activites with attention. Pay exquisite attention to tying your shoes. What are your fingers doing? How do the laces feel in your hands? How much pressure do they exert when you tug on them?

Create a New Track Record

About once a month set aside about twice as much material to work on or study as you would ordinarily tackle in one evening. Then work on it intensively until you finish. For instance, you might complete an essay on the civil rights movement a week before it's due. Keep this deadline, even if it means staying up late. Usually we don't encourage all-nighters or even too many late nights, but this exercise, this stretch, will increase your capacity to accomplish things through focused efforts.

Making promises and keeping them are fundamental to lasting change and real achievement. If you do not keep your word, you do not consider yourself reliable and you will not take your own statements seriously. This weakens you. Perhaps you have already weakened yourself in just this way by not keeping deadlines or by breaking promises to yourself. Use this exercise to create a new track record.

Create New Operating Instructions

Rather than wishing yourself luck with your personal change, take another key step to ensure your success: Create precise internal instructions for using a new behavior you wish to make habitual. Then practice it until it becomes overlearned—a term psychologists use for a behavior so well rehearsed that it becomes automatic. The first step is to find a typical situation in which you used the old behavior and find a new, specific behavior to replace it.

Say you want to become more patient. Perhaps whenever the line for dropping a course is too long or all the dryers in the laundry room are busy, you typically bolt, losing the time you already devoted to the task and failing to complete your task.

Imagine this situation, see yourself in it, and then, at the point at which your impatience formerly overwhelmed you, find a new behavior to substitute for leaving. Consider as many possibilities as you want before coming up with this new behavior. You might decide to work on a list of Spanish verbs you want to memorize or a book of Sudoku puzzles.

However, this solution depends on carrying one or both items. If you don't do so regularly, you will have to learn a new habit in addition to the new behavior. It's not that hard to learn the additional step, and it may be worthwhile if you spend a lot of time in lines. Whipping out a verb list or puzzle would certainly force you to rethink fuming and leaving.

A new behavior that doesn't involve anything external might be even better. You might decide that whenever you are forced to wait, you will recite your favorite poetry or song lyrics to yourself or do various visualizations. Or you could think of these as a backup in case you forget the verbs or puzzles.

When you come up with a new behavioral choice, develop an internal instruction to tie the new behavior to a specific triggering event. A trigger can be either the event that prompted the old behavior or the event you want to associate with the new behavior. Standing in a slow-moving line used to trigger your impatience. For your new behavior, the triggering event must be one that will occur reliably enough to bring out the new behavior.

Put your new specific operating instruction in the following form: "Whenever I stand in any line, I will *always*...." Then insert the behavior you decide will work best for you. If you choose the Spanish verbs, the sentence would end "pull out my list of Spanish verbs and begin to memorize them." Note the use of the word *always* in the instructions. Always use *always* in your specific operating instructions.

You must also develop a specific operating instruction to see that you always carry your Spanish verb list. This would be, "Whenever I pick up my keys, I put the Spanish verb list in my pocket." Keep the verb list in the same place as your keys.

It is important to work with your new specific operating instructions when you are not in the situation and to keep working with them whether you encounter success or failure in the actual situation. You will experience a particular pleasure when you employ the new behavior in a real situation, which is all to the good. Your goal, however, is to make the new behavior become your automatic response. Repetition is the key to achieving this outcome.

Do It Again—and Again and Again

If you took music lessons as a child, you may have groaned every time you had to play scales. If you stuck with it, however, you may have come to love what you might have hated at first. Repetition is necessary to learn and to lock in any new behavior—to lock in change. So learn to love it.

You need *many* repetitions of any new behavior to overlearn it and make it automatic. For the best results, rehearse a new behavior consistently when you are cool and unflustered. This will help you internalize the instructions and become mentally accustomed to the new choice.

At the minimum, repeat your new specific operating instructions five times in the morning and five times in the evening. After you complete each set of repetitions, add the statement, "I will follow these instructions carefully." Finish by visualizing yourself doing each new behavior.

Continue this exercise indefinitely but for at least one month after you notice that you are consistently using a new behavioral change, such as making new food choices or employing new study habits.

JOURNALING ASSIGNMENT : Making It Real

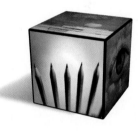

Practice your new behaviors in real life. Each day create as many opportunities as possible in which to use your new instructions, including simulations. For instance, seek out long lines, stand in them, and use your new substitute behaviors. When you are about to enter the situation, repeat the instructions and visualize the new behavior. Nothing increases the speed at which you adopt new behaviors like rehearsal in real life.

Keep track of how often you follow your new operating instructions in your journal. Notice how quickly they become automatic.

Check the Warning Labels on Risky Behavior

On the packages of certain medications, you see black boxes that draw attention to serious, sometimes life-threatening risks associated with their use. Depending on the message and your health history, you might decide that the possible risks outweigh the potential benefits of the drug. Some behaviors also pose such serious risks that you should probably think of them as carrying a black-box warning.

Specific operating instructions are especially useful for curbing unnecessarily risky behavior. If you have taken unnecessary risks in the past with your health or safety—binge drinking, for instance, or not consistently using condoms if you are sexually active—you need to make new choices that are healthier for you. Once you have chosen to eliminate the risky behavior, you can make the new healthier choice automatic by following the steps we described earlier. (See the "Don't Go There" lab in the *Labs for An Invitation to Personal Change*.)

Value yourself and your health enough to make decisions about risky behavior after cool and lengthy reflection. Decide on the best course for you, and determine exactly what you *will do* instead of what you *have done* in the past. Then create specific operating instructions and practice the instructions plus the new behavior until that behavior becomes automatic in real time.

Check the Box

Know which activities are black-box activities for you to avoid. Heavy partying? Smoking pot? Online gambling? You may already know which ones you should steer clear of but might not have known how to avoid them. Now you know better and you can do better. Set yourself up for a specific, healthier, alternative behavior in the future.

Knowing how to eliminate and replace risky behavior increases your luck by eliminating unlucky behavior. As you gain ever-increasing mastery, you will unmistakably feel your ability to influence and change the direction of your life through your own actions.

Welcome to the director's chair.

Reaching Out

Joining forces with others changes everything—including personal change. Merely being around others—a person or a group of people—affects behavior. The first social psychology experiment simply measured the speed at which volunteers reeled in fishing line when alone versus when with others. The result: People reeled faster in the presence of even one other person.

As subsequent studies have shown, runners speed up when they jog together (or even when they run past someone who might be looking at them). Dieters who team with support partners lose more weight than those who diet alone. Women with advanced breast cancer live longer when they participate in support groups.

Only you can choose to direct personal change in your life. But you don't have to go it alone. As you launch your master plan for personal change, reach out to a carefully selected friend, partner, buddy, coach, mentor, colleague, support group, or online community. Having someone at your side, urging you on or backing you up when you face discouragement, can make a crucial difference in successful change.

This chapter shows you how to talk with others about change, find an accountability partner, and take full advantage of the power of groups of advisers and experts who have information you need.

Why People Need People

The more serious your goal or project, the more you will benefit from support. Mildly daunting things like personal change are easier to tackle with a support system in place. Having company on your journey isn't an expression of weakness or dependency but a matter of having backup when you need it. Knowing why you can use assistance and being able to ask for it are signs of mature independence. Would you climb Mount Everest alone? (See the "Help Yourself" lab in the *Labs for An Invitation to Personal Change.*)

The right sort of involvement helps you move further faster and with better results. Athletes, like competitive cyclists, know they can accomplish more when they train with others. Rock stars have posses. NASCAR and Formula One drivers have pit crews. Politicians have aides and advisers.

The most widely used form of psychotherapy today is group therapy. As rigorous studies have shown, groups are especially effective because they provide a safe and supportive environment in which members can share and discuss their problems, hear alternative ways to solve them, learn from the experiences of others, and discover new ways of interacting. You don't have to join a therapy group to change, but support can be crucial for your change efforts.

At the minimum we recommend that you find one person to check in with at least weekly to support you and help keep you accountable to your goals. This person—part pal, part shoulder to lean on, part guru—is a key player on your team. In addition, gather as you need them other people whose personal experience, expertise, or knowledge can help you anticipate challenges you may face and plan how to deal with them. They might include professors or instructors who have inside information related to your long-range goals and who have advice on pathways to seek and to avoid.

JOURNALING ASSIGNMENT : Whom Do You Need?

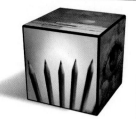

1. Spend some time considering the type of support you could best use and whom you could enlist to accompany you while you change. What roles do you want this person to play—witness, monitor, coach, personal trainer, cheerleader, confidante, boot camp sergeant, or all of the above? Make a list of your needs and wishes and the qualities you think would help you most. At a minimum, your objective should be to find someone who can aid you in staying on track and nudge you when you reach a plateau or become distracted, discouraged, or otherwise tempted to throw in the towel.

_____

_____

_____

_____

_____

_____

_____

_____

_____

_____

_____

_____

2. Jot down the names of potential candidates, and audition them in your mind.

_____

_____

_____

_____

_____

_____

_____

_____

_____

_____

_____

Be brutally honest. Do you want to turn your best friend into the nutrition police? Would you resent your roommate nagging you to get your work done on time? The person you choose not only should be trustworthy and neutral but also should have no personal stake in the outcome other than wanting the best for you. This eliminates family members, spouses, boyfriends, and girlfriends. They play other roles in your life that could create conflicts of interest or other complications.

Above all, you must respect your change partner. Beware of rescuers and people who have a high need to control. You can usually tell who they are because right away they want to tell you what to do and when and how to do it. Your support persons must work in service of your goals and play the role you ask them to play. This role may change from time to time, but you are the one who calls the shots.

Choosing a Change Partner

Don't get bogged down looking for the perfect person. However, if you feel hesitant about asking someone, you may have a good reason. Trust your intuition. When you are reasonably sure you have the right person in mind, think about it before going to bed and literally sleep on it. If you still feel you have the right person the next morning, wait one more day to ask.

Since change is your decision, you can choose not to talk to your support person about the specifics of your goals at first or you can go into as much detail as you choose. It's your call. If you'd rather not reveal all the details of your goals, that's fine. You can just check in with your change partner regularly about your progress. You can always talk more openly later—if and when you feel more comfortable.

If you prefer to begin even less directly, you might just have coffee with one or two people you find supportive. Talk in general ways about goals and change to see how it feels to have such a discussion and where it might lead.

Before your partner accepts, the two of you need to reach an understanding about how you want him or her to play this role. Keep the relationship and the demands on the other person straightforward and simple. Do not request an open-ended or long-term commitment. Although it can be beneficial, you don't have to have the same change partner throughout your entire campaign.

Keep in mind that your success is your responsibility, not your change partner's. If you ask this person to prod or be firm with you, don't be resentful when he or she does so.

If your top candidate turns down your request, accept the refusal as the best outcome for both of you. You wouldn't do well with someone who doesn't want to take the role for whatever reason. You will find other support, so don't feel your success depends on one particular person.

▶ Buddy Up

Rather than looking for a support partner, consider being a buddy with someone else making changes so that you can coach and encourage each other. This works as long as you are both equally committed to change and you avoid competition. If you find a possible change buddy, arrange a trial "marriage" for about a month. Then you can review the arrangement and decide whether to continue.

Using a Change Partner

Start simply, and limit the arrangement. Meet to discuss your joint expectations, and go over your plan in as much detail as seems appropriate to you. After this, check in regularly (weekly is usually best), report your progress on specific goals and tasks, and set goals for the next check-in.

If you feel discouraged between check-ins, call your support person. As you both become more comfortable with this partnership, you can tailor and refine the process of receiving support. The goal is to keep you moving and on target. If you feel stuck, ask your partner for suggestions.

Recruiting the Rest of Your Change Team

It takes a team to launch a new business, compete in a relay race, or win a pennant. We suggest that you put together a dream team of your own to support your personal change campaign. Think of people from whom you can learn. When the time seems right, sound them out about sharing their information or skills. Again, you don't have to inform these people of your overall plan or even tell them that they are a part of your team. For your purposes, a quick summary may be enough. On the other hand, you may be ready to tell all. You decide how much you want to reveal.

If a major part of your change efforts relates to future career possibilities, you may look for someone who can mentor you or arrange for you to shadow him or her. Shadowing—observing someone working and taking notes on what you observe—allows you to see firsthand how that person reacts and thinks. At the same time, you gain the opportunity to absorb subtle intangibles such as attitude, pace, and the "feel" of the activity as the person carries it out. Before someone agrees to this, however, he or she may need more information about what you hope to accomplish.

Through the process of recruiting team members, you may discover someone who provides unexpected assistance and you may move in unanticipated directions. If gathering information requires talking to people you don't know, ask your contacts for names of others who would be willing to talk with you. Interviewing a friend of a friend can be an easier first step to change than trying to go it alone. You will quickly compile a series of leads. Even if you obtain only one name, this person may give you additional contacts and invaluable information.

You have resources at your fingertips that you may have overlooked. Open yourself to these possibilities. What about a former camp counselor, an ex-boss, a Sunday School teacher, your priest or rabbi, another veteran, or a high school coach who might love to help an alum? Who else might give you an encouraging lift and provide you with knowledge gained from personal experience?

Do not overlook the resource of teacher's assistants and upperclassmen, especially ones in your major. What about the people who led your college orientation or the resident advisors in your dorm? Your school may have a center that provides career advice and brief personal counseling. If you want someone neutral with whom to sort out a personal decision, you need look no further.

Prep Yourself

Before each meeting with anyone from your change team, visualize the meeting in detail, including as much vivid sensory material as possible. See the situation and smell, sense, see, hear, and even taste as many specifics as you can. Then imagine the course of the conversation. See yourself asking good questions that provide valuable information. Finally, sense the appreciation you feel and express for what you learn.

JOURNALING ASSIGNMENT : Log on for Virtual Support

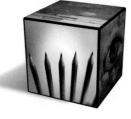

Every month millions of Americans log on to websites targeted to individuals dealing with stress, weight problems, smoking, mental disorders, addictions, chronic illnesses, and a host of other problems. Why? Online support is convenient, anonymous, and available around the clock.

Search the Internet for websites related to the behaviors you want to change or the habits you wish to create. Make a list of the most useful sites, which might include blogs, bulletin boards, chat groups, and web pages created by professional organizations or commercial sponsors.

Preparing Others for Your Change

Your support team can help you with an important task: how to talk to others about changes you intend to make. They can also support you in preparing for occasional unexpected or unpleasant reactions.

You may have been thinking about and quietly preparing for change for weeks or months. As you go public with your change, people will inevitably begin to notice. Some will celebrate your decisions and progress, especially those who truly care about you and your well-being. They may see you as a role model and welcome your changes as an impetus to make similar changes of their own. A few people will approve of anything you propose because they like you or want you to like them.

However, not everyone will be happy about your changes, and some of their reactions could cause problems. Some people may feel threatened because what you are changing draws attention to something they feel they also should change but have not. Others may disapprove because they dismiss anything out of the ordinary as threatening to them. Still others may not grant approval without wanting to know more than you may prefer to reveal.

You may or may not be able to predict from your past experiences which friends will respond in which way. The people closest to you—family, friends, roommates, coworkers—know your routines, which they see as normal, and they expect you to follow them.

Say you spend hours every weekend playing cards or shopping with your pals. If you decide to join a choir or band, you'll have to practice instead. Your friends may feel slighted and discourage you from your plan. "What's the matter with you?" they may ask. "Don't you have time for us anymore?"

If you radically change your study habits, you may get similar reactions from those who know they too should change but who have not yet made the commitment. Head off such potentially awkward situations by telling the people around you—particularly those you live with—any changes that might affect them.

"You're Perfect Just the Way You Are"

Be prepared for another kind of response that can be much trickier. Some people may feel that you want them to tell you that you are wonderful the way you are and that you do not need to change. They may mean it and say it because they genuinely care for you. Under ordinary circumstances, you would savor such unconditional approval. However, if you have not yet committed yourself fully to change, the suggestion that you don't have to change may reinforce any ambivalence you feel. Just stay in the director's chair. Breathe.

As you change, be sure not to abandon legitimate responsibilities to others, which could annoy people accustomed to relying on you. Change does not require becoming self-absorbed and ignoring reasonable demands on your time. You still have to show up at floor meetings or take out the garbage when it's your turn. If you need to make adjustments, talk them over openly to arrive at workable solutions. If you can't participate in every rush activity at your fraternity or sorority, for instance, give advance notice and make clear what you can and will do. If you want to spend more time with your children, explain to your boss why you're turning down extra shifts.

If you take these steps and don't receive support, get whatever help you need from those supporting you and simply address the problem again. Issues about expectations and responsibilities often require repeated discussion. Call an open meeting with your housemates, if need be, and keep working toward a solution. Your friends or family may not realize how deeply committed you are to a particular personal change.

Because you don't want negative reactions to swamp your boat, be careful about *how* you talk about the specific changes you intend to make and be selective about whom you choose to tell. Each time you talk to someone about your plan to change, you momentarily become somewhat vulnerable to that person's response. Pay especially close attention to—and rein in—the sense that you must explain yourself. Stay in the director's chair. This is your movie. When you feel that you have to justify what you're doing, you are implicitly asking for approval of your plan and of your decision to follow it. People respond accordingly, and you begin to lose precious degrees of control that you need to succeed.

Our advice: Avoid seeking approval. Why put someone else in charge, even briefly?

Keep what you say to others simple. This too might provoke some negative responses, but it doesn't necessarily mean that a person no longer likes and values you. Since people's reactions can potentially weaken your resolve to change—particularly before you have made an absolute decision to go forward—stay focused on your intention for telling. You are not seeking approval. Your goal is to inform those who may need to know and those who, by knowing in advance, may make your change easier to actualize.

Remember: The decision to change is yours. Never put it in someone else's hands. You also decide whom you will talk to and how much you will reveal. You don't want to give away too much of the plot.

real change: tomorrow is another diet (continued)

The moment of truth for Jessica, whom you met on page 34 of Chapter 3, came when she could no longer zip up any of the jeans in her closet. She had to rummage around for a pair of sweats, her "fat pants," as her mother called them. Jessica didn't want to repeat her high school pattern of starving herself for weeks and then gaining back the weight she'd lost—and then some. But Jessica also realized another truth about herself: She could use some help.

By scanning the bulletin boards at the student union, Jessica found a variety of weight loss groups on campus. One called F.A.T. (for Fit and Trim) appealed to her because she liked the idea of group exercise classes, bike rides, and weekend fun runs. While working out together, she became friendly with Janeel, who also wanted to lose weight sensibly and safely. The two became diet buddies.

When their dormmates would call for a pizza, Jessica and Janeel would get together for a walk or go to the gym. Whenever their schedules allowed, they'd eat meals together. When one reached for a chocolate chip cookie or some pie, the other would gently ask, "Are you sure you want to do that?"

Jessica was excited when she could fit into her jeans again. But she is even more delighted by how strong and energetic she feels—and by the new friendship she's forged with Janeel.

Shock Absorption

After weeks or months of contemplating, planning, and preparing, you take off. You can practically feel yourself changing, and you revel in the thrill of your new adventure. Maybe you're so pumped that you're sure nothing can stop you.

Then you come down with the flu. Or you see on Facebook that your ex is in a new committed relationship. Or you find out that your cat was hit by a car. To top it off, the changes you've made may no longer feel so exhilarating. While everyone else in Pilates class arcs into a plow, you can't get your hips off the mat. You forget the apple that was supposed to keep you from craving a candy bar midafternoon. Or your friends are giving you a hard time for not wanting to play beer pong anymore.

We've warned you that there would be days like this. Be happy and enjoy it when things are going well—but realize the honeymoon isn't necessarily going to last forever.

As you power toward your personal change goals, you naturally encounter surprises, roadblocks, detours, and delays. Of course, you ran into obstacles when you were living your old life, but now that you're in the process of directing change, they may hit you harder, particularly if you are not ready. You may be a little more vulnerable because you're enthusiastically developing new skills and trying out new experiences. It's okay to say "Ouch!"—just don't decide to interpret a bump in the road as evidence that you were not really making progress or that you're back to same old, same old.

We can't prevent rough patches or protect you from disappointments, but we can offer you something more useful: shock absorbers. The techniques and strategies described in this chapter are designed to increase your ability to resist the slings and arrows of outrageous fortune and bounce back from setbacks.

Think for a minute about this word. A *setback* is something that sets you back some. In your life to date, temporary setbacks have undoubtedly accompanied all progress you have made. *Temporary* is the key word. You are the one who decides whether you will allow any setback to become a reason to stop moving forward.

For the rest of your life the techniques in this chapter can keep you on track and help you refocus where you're going by redirecting you to the goals you value most. They will help you swerve around some common roadblocks and steer toward your deepest values. And if you do spin out and wind up in the weeds, we'll tell you what to do about that, too.

Staying on Track

Did you ever go to the beach and, after playing in the surf for a while, discover that you were a considerable distance down the beach from your towel? The reason? Under the influence of wind and current, you drifted. During your change effort, without noticing exactly when or how it happened, you may find you are somewhere different from where you intended to be.

Change, like the pursuit of any new path, carries this risk. When you head into unexplored territory, you no longer have the comfort of familiar signposts. Merely by taking your eyes off the goal or becoming distracted, you can veer off a little. Stray an inch off course and, if you do not correct, after a few miles you have some distance to cover in order to get back to where you want to be.

Staying on track while new things are happening requires knowing what needs to be done and keeping it in front of you at all times. The following assignments can help.

JOURNALING ASSIGNMENT : Check Your GPS: Where Are You Now?

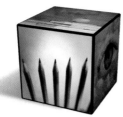

You can go off course by delaying starting (aka procrastinating) or by getting distracted and not finishing what you intended to complete. If you know or suspect you may have drifted, check your bearings. Go back to Chapter 4, read what you wrote, and then ask yourself the following questions. Write the answers in your *Journal for An Invitation to Personal Change* or in the space that follows.

1. Where were you intending to go when you started out?

    _____

    _____

    _____

    _____

    _____

    _____

    _____

2. What was your aim?

    _____

    _____

    _____

    _____

    _____

    _____

    _____

3. Is it still the same?

    _____

    _____

    _____

    _____

    _____

    _____

    _____

4. What is the shortest or best route to....?

_____

_____

_____

_____

_____

_____

_____

_____

5. What support do I need to get back on track?

_____

_____

_____

_____

_____

_____

_____

_____

After taking stock, reaffirm your personal change goal. If you discover that you have merely drifted, retrace your steps and get going again. If you are having trouble making your new behavior fit your former self-concept, take a breather. Realize that it takes some time to expand the concept of who we think we are so that it encompasses our new behaviors.

Your reappraisal might reveal a change in your long-term goals. Say you've rediscovered your love of working with young children and decide to switch your major from business to early childhood education. If so, begin activities in line with this new revised goal. Reach out to counselors, mentors, friends, and experts. Check the academic requirements. Look into internship opportunities. Talk to teachers in local preschools and kindergartens.

Realign everything in your life to be in harmony with and support your path. Concentrate on actions that best and most efficiently serve your new objective and get results. Load up on education prerequisites and requirements. Volunteer in a church or after-school child-care program. When you sit down to study every day, keep in mind that you are not just studying for a course but also preparing for a career that will bring you gratification and joy.

You will soon be on track again, even though you're headed in a new direction.

Strengthening Your Shock Absorbers

Locking in a major change can take a while, sometimes longer than an academic quarter or semester. During this time—usually about six months—you can experience an array of feelings. The satisfaction of directing change can continue to provide motivation, force, and energy. But what was exciting at first can become somewhat more routine. If you know this can happen, you are partially prepared. However, there is more you can do.

Every chapter in this section is designed to build skills that increase your sense of mastery and efficacy and help you know that you can direct and maintain change. Developing patience and persistence, learning to tolerate frustration, creating an overview of where you are going, and identifying goals all prepare you to be your own agent of change. If you strengthen your focus and your resolve, you can indeed become a force.

But setbacks by their very nature throw you off. So here are other things that research shows can anchor you and increase your stability and shock resistance:

- Pleasure
- Physical health
- A form of spiritual practice, formally religious or not
- Faith and a belief in a higher power
- Prayer
- Regular meditation and other attention-focusing practices
- Art, literature, music, and dance
- Appropriate sleep and rest
- A healthy diet
- A strong sense of ethics
- At least one close friend or a circle of friends
- Good physical and mental health practices
- Fun
- A sense of humor
- A sense of following a path with meaning
- Work that is intrinsically satisfying
- Other intrinsically satisfying activities
- A sense of gratitude
- A practice of contemplating what you have to be grateful for
- A larger view of what is important beyond self-interest
- An awareness of and appreciation for life

Even with considerable inner reserves and advance planning, you may lose your footing. Whatever you do, do not consider any stumble a failure. The only failure will be failing to mine the situation to discover as much information as you can. Mistakes and setbacks teach exactly what you need to move forward—especially if you think you have hit a wall or crashed and burned.

Do a postmortem on this little episode. Then regroup, reload, and launch Plan B. Avoid drama. Consider all of this as nothing more than a midcourse correction. When you drive, you make hundreds of tiny course corrections in order to travel in a straight line. It is the same with change. Sometimes when you're driving, you come to a detour. This is the same with change.

JOURNALING ASSIGNMENT : Your Best Mistake

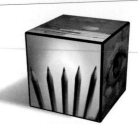

Describe a mistake you made or setback you've experienced in the space that follows. Then note what you learned from handling this setback, what strengths and strategies helped you through it, what you adjusted, and how much stronger you are for overcoming it.

_____

_____

_____

_____

_____

_____

_____

_____

_____

_____

_____

_____

Block Your Escape Routes

Nearly all rough patches, obstacles, and setbacks provide one dangerously addictive possibility: the chance for a self-indulgent escape from the whole change project. Think back. Have you set change goals in the past but quit before achieving them because you ran into a rough patch?

If so, when the going gets difficult, you may again be tempted to take some well-trod escape routes. You may already know what they are because you have used them so often. Do you veg out, overeat, drink, take drugs, procrastinate, hook up, or go to bed and pull the blankets over your head?

List some escape routes you've tried in the past—and where they've led.

_____

_____

_____

_____

_____

_____

_____

_____

Escape "works" only in the sense that it provides immediate although short-lived relief from anxiety. This relief is its seduction—what makes escape tempting. As an actual solution, escape is a complete failure. The only way to get over or around any difficult situation is to go *through* it—go right into the teeth of it and learn from it.

Resist temptation to make small obstacles big in order to justify quitting and not changing. Would you abandon your car if you lost the keys? Drop out of school because you blew a test? Of course not. If you indulge in self-pity when you confront obstacles now, you could be running for the exits before you know it.

No Failure to Fear

As we've said before and will say again, the biggest obstacle to change is fear of failure. This fear prompts you to step away from risks, including the risks of personal change, and look for a way out. But escape includes more downside risks than the failure you fear.

A life well lived is marked by one failure after another. This is nothing to mourn or evade. You must embrace this reality to begin the journey toward a real life. Only by taking risks and experiencing failure can you gain sufficient knowledge to learn how to live.

Learning and changing involve failure. If you have always accomplished whatever you set out to do with ease and without failure, either your ambitions are modest or you have confined yourself to familiar territory. If your primary objective is to avoid failure, you put an immediate lid on how far you can go.

You write your autobiography daily, moment to moment. If you do not take risks into account, you will not survive. If you make evading risks your only concern, you will miss opportunities. Failures are exactly the opportunities you need. And you need as many as it takes to grow accustomed to thinking this way.

The inventor Thomas Edison systematically tried more than 16,000 materials in search of a filament for what he hoped would be an electrical source of light. Only after 16,000 failures did he find one—tungsten—that worked. Learn to consider failure the ore from which you extract success, because failure is a richer source of information and enlightenment than quick success.

The only way to deal with fear of failure is head on. When your idea of what constitutes success and failure changes, your fear of failure dissipates. The only real failure you will ever experience is not to begin. Pursuing your heart's desire with unquenchable effort is worth doing whether or not you succeed. The real achievement in life is to participate instead of hanging back.

Failure is nothing more than evidence that you are learning something new—unless you make it more. You decide when to consider a failure a learning experience and when to call the entire change effort a failure. Our opinion is that the only two things to run from are characterizing a setback as a failure of the change effort or calling yourself a failure for experiencing one. And our idea of failure? Hanging back and avoiding or quitting.

Everything else is just part of the learning process. Remember your first time on a snowboard or first try at an omelet? You probably weren't a natural at either. Absence of failure is often evidence of sticking to the tried-and-true—and quite possibly boring—safety of no risks.

Keep running your show. Take the bad with the good. Do not abandon your role or your change campaign. When you duck out of your rightful position in the director's chair, others feel compelled to step in and take over. If you operate from an "I'll fumble around and see if someone notices and bails me out" position, you set yourself up for a life of remaining dependent on others or for future struggles to regain the control you relinquish. In the meantime, you fall behind and lose time while people draw potentially damaging conclusions about you. You also may draw some damning conclusions about yourself.

If the idea of escape tantalizes you, turn to your accountability partner or seek encouragement from your support circle. If need be, go to the counseling center on campus and talk with someone about any ways in which your behavior is sabotaging your success. Be careful about this, however, because you can fall into using counseling—a great tool—as an excuse for not moving forward. If you decide you must resolve menacing psychological issues before you can make personal changes, you only lose time.

Are You Getting in Your Own Way?

You may not even be aware of any tendency to trip over your own feet until you start to change. Because you consider whatever you habitually do as normal, you may have accepted self-defeating behavior, not as a choice but as simply the way you are. In fact, you made many choices in the process of becoming who you "naturally" are. Everything that feels normal and natural now was once a matter of choice and in the beginning felt awkward and new. When you can recognize this element of choice, you have the opportunity to make a new one.

Try the following simple exercise: Take off your wristwatch, and place it on the other wrist. Leave it there for a day. Notice whether it feels unnatural or odd and whether this feeling changes.

Of course, there isn't anything "natural" about wearing your watch on one wrist or the other. It's simply a matter of choice—like the way you shave or apply moisturizer. You always do these things the same way. Change them, and notice how you feel. The point isn't to throw yourself off but to show that you can continue unhelpful or pointless habits because they feel "normal" and balk at very useful changes because they feel strange at first.

If even simple changes can unsettle you, how will you fulfill your potential or accomplish a life choice or a dream? Small patterns migrate from specific situations and grow into big, generalized patterns until you come to view a set of habits as who you fundamentally are. If you see that you haven't persisted, for instance, you may conclude that you lack persistence and that you can't finish things you start. If you see that you avoid things, you come to think that you are a coward.

Say you are putting off filing the final part of your application for study abroad. Avoiding the paperwork may seem a small thing. But focus on the following: What is it you fear about reaching your goal? New demands to live up to? New expectations from others? The unknown challenges of spending time in a foreign country? Disappointment if you aren't accepted? Figure it out, because if you delay, you create a new problem—avoiding. Then, by not solving the tendency to avoid, you make the stakes higher still.

As you analyze ways in which you may be tripping yourself up, keep another thing in mind. If you have not reached a change goal as rapidly as you wanted, do not try to save face by quitting. Otherwise, after all your hard work, you will pull away from the struggle before you reach the rewards.

Achieving any important, satisfying goal takes time. If you sign on only for what is immediately fun and easy, you shrink your life down to a limited range of shallow activities and interests and block yourself from making changes that would set you free. And you never find out what it's like to spend a semester in Rio studying Portuguese.

▶ ## *Twice as Hard*

Picture yourself redoubling your current level of intensity and effort. See, in specific detail, what this would mean to your current efforts. In which areas would you strengthen your resolve? How would you become relentless in pursuit of your objectives?

Repeat this exercise daily for at least 10 days or until you feel yourself solidly back on track.

Are You (Were You) Ready to Grow Up?

The biggest change you will ever make is the change from adolescence to adulthood. You're either in this transition now or you remember it well. You make this change in stages over a long time. Learning what your goals are and discovering how you want to direct your life story from this point forward are crucial parts of becoming grownup.

Throughout your life, your parents may have inspired you and showered you with good advice. They may have encouraged you to make any number of choices with which you are deeply content. They may continue to provide support both materially and through their wisdom and goodwill. Nonetheless, at some point your life becomes yours and yours alone to direct—not your parents' and not your partner's.

There is no single moment when the apprenticeship of childhood ends and adulthood officially begins. Sometimes circumstances—war, poverty, and violence—propel youngsters into adulthood far too soon. Other young people postpone the final steps of growing up for as long as possible. In the grownup (or maybe not so grownup) equivalent of a kid on the high dive at summer camp, they get all the way to the edge then inch backward rather than jump off.

You probably know people who have done this. Remember the slackers in high school who ended up taking a fifth or "bridge" year before starting college? Other students transfer from one college to another, often leaving one school so abruptly they don't accumulate any credits. Then there are the undecideds who postpone choosing a major or dabble in so many fields that they need an extra year or two to graduate.

What's wrong with dragging your feet on the way to adulthood? Why not remain a student as long as you can? After all, college is a safe haven, a way station for intellectual and social experimentation. You're surrounded by vibrant, intelligent, attractive people. You set your own hours. You can pick and choose from an array of pleasant activities. Others may prepare your meals and tend to your well-being. Even if you live at home and commute, you have special status as a college student. Sure, you have classes, papers, midterms, grades—all demanding but not quite adult expectations.

But if you are postponing the step into adult freedom and adult responsibility, you are stopping yourself from directing the changes you need to make to achieve your goals and reach your full measure of accomplishment. Look inside. You will know whether you are postponing, balking, avoiding, or genuinely exploring alternatives. Each feels different.

You control the choices you make about your change goals. If you delay choosing your goals and cling to the idea that you have others to please or appease, this will register in you as a sense of unease. And you will arrange secretly to trip yourself up in the pursuit of goals you didn't choose for yourself.

The extended vacation of college provides you with plenty of wiggle room but ultimately no escape. There also is no evading other major life transitions, like a loved one's illness or death, a job loss, parenthood, or a suddenly empty nest. At every life passage you may withdraw briefly to question yourself and your readiness. No matter the circumstance or transition, the formula for growth is the same: Plunge into the next phase of the school-of-life curriculum and learn from it everything you can.

Whose Goals Are You Pursuing?

Are you a premed student because your mother never had the chance to fulfill her dream of becoming a doctor? Are you going out for lacrosse because your brother was a college all-star? Are you trying one major after another because you would rather train to be a paramedic than get a degree in liberal arts? Are you taking evening courses because your supervisor suggested them or because you want to move into management?

In your journal, list each change goal you have created. For each one, examine the source and inspiration for the particular goal. (There is nothing wrong if the inspiration came from someone other than you.)

Give each goal a rating from 0 to 100 for the degree to which the goal is one you embrace as your own, using 0 for one that you do not embrace at all and 100 for a goal fully embraced by you. Make a second rating to express the importance of accomplishing each goal, using 0 for a goal completely unimportant to you and 100 for one as important as you could imagine.

Now make some additional notes about what you have learned from this journaling exercise.

Backup Your Backups

On your way to new habits, you need backup support at every turn. Developing Plan B in case Plan A fails isn't enough. You need Plan C, too. Your best backups grow from your own experience. Let's say that when you got stressed or anxious in the past you usually dropped projects and forgot about them for weeks at a time. You decide that as a backup you will call your support partner as soon as that kind of frustration starts to build.

What if you can't reach this person? This is a critical moment. Without another backup plan, you are at risk. You need multiple rehearsed backup strategies in place in case the first one fails. Don't imagine you will stay cool and come up with a plan on the spot. Improvising opens the gates for old, automatic behavior patterns, such as fleeing the situation. Know your next steps in advance.

In this case, you might develop specific operating instructions about how to talk yourself down to a calmer state. You could focus your attention on your breathing and count your breaths. Or you could visualize a favorite tranquil place—a beach, say, or a garden—that you associate with relaxation and well-being. You could count backward from a hundred. Once you compose yourself, you could resolve to take up where you left off with renewed energy.

If you do not know in advance what to do when you hit an obstacle or bumpy patch on the way to personal change, you are more likely to waffle and, as a consequence, head in the direction of quitting. If, instead, you calmly survey the situation, make midcourse corrections, and rejoin the battle more fully, you hugely increase your chances of success.

The key is you. No other person holds the answer; nothing else can lead you where you want to go. No one is always there or can take better care of you than you. You have abundant internal resources you can develop and turn to in tough times. Go inward, connect with your strength, be your own lifeline, and regain your footing.

Relapse Rehearsals

Since setbacks, lapses, and even dreaded relapses come with the territory of personal change, you need to recognize them for what they are: brief sidetracks into old, deeply carved behaviors that, if not caught quickly, automatically lead to other dead ends. Therapists who help individuals, families, and groups deal with unhealthy behavior such as addictions have developed specific techniques to lower the likelihood of relapses. One of the most powerful is rehearsal.

How does a recovering alcoholic get ready for a Super Bowl party? Can a problem gambler survive a night in Las Vegas without blowing a wad of money? How will a dieter stick to a weight loss plan over the holidays? All can prepare for these challenging situations and prevent relapses by rehearing their new behavior.

The ex-drinker can begin with new operating instructions, such as "Whenever I am at any party where alcohol is available, I always drink fruit juice, sparkling water, or another nonalcoholic beverage." Beyond this, the ex-drinker not only mentally plays out a step-by-step approach to dealing with friends on Super Bowl Sunday but also practices standing around chatting with a nonlethal drink in hand. The ex-gambler who plans to be in Vegas for a car show imagines walking past the bright lights and dark poker rooms of the casinos and actually, not just in fantasy, walks by them without pausing or entering. The dieter visualizes politely declining whipped cream for Grandma's pecan pie and eating just three bites and practices this scenario.

Through mental rehearsals and role-play simulations, people develop the specific coping skills they need to avoid temptation. Rehearsal reduces the likelihood of a relapse, as well as the length and seriousness of any that might occur.

The following exercise can help you rehearse your way around a potential relapse.

▶ Dress Rehearsal

Think of the situation most likely to lead to a setback or relapse. Visualize yourself in the scene. Listen to someone who is offering you a drug, drink, or decadently rich dessert— whatever you've pledged to avoid. Feel the temptation of staying in your snug and cozy bed on a cold morning instead of getting up for the early run you'd planned. See yourself tempted by a friend's offer of a ticket to that night's basketball game when you should be studying for a midterm.

Then, in vivid detail, visualize yourself just saying no, getting up and pulling on your sweats with a smile on your face, or turning down the invitation for the basketball game because the wiser part of your mind prevails. Then do an actual dress rehearsal, a role play of each of these situations in detail with friends from your support circle.

Building Resiliency

When a tornado or flood wipes out an entire town, some people suffer only minor damage to their homes but pack up and move to safer ground. Others lose everything but are determined to rebuild. Why are some individuals crushed by a disaster while others are able to cope and carry on with their lives?

From extensive studies of survivors of all sorts of traumas, psychologists have identified common characteristics of those who bounce back from serious setbacks. Resilient people typically

- are resourceful
- believe that they have a right to survive and thrive
- are able to attract and use support
- extract the maximum benefit from the support they receive
- keep in mind images of figures who have provided support in the past
- are flexible
- have goals
- embody an indomitable fighting spirit
- tend to make positive statements

In the face of a crisis, resilient people turn right back into adversity and feed off it as a source of energy. Instead of allowing external events or circumstances to crush them, they choose to draw inspiration and renewed force from the very extremity of the situation they confront. The resilient not only do not allow themselves to be defeated but do not even entertain such thoughts. Instead, they learn from challenges and thrive on responding to them. And over time they respond better, faster, and more effectively.

How do you compare with the resilient individuals we've described? At first glance they may seem larger than life, more heroic and courageous than you can imagine being. But rest assured that they were not born this way. Like other behaviors, resiliency can be acquired and developed. *You* can make yourself more resilient.

The first step is a purposeful decision to interpret obstacles as challenges and as a source of lessons. Simply make the conscious choice to see setbacks and hardships in this way. Then decide that nothing will crush you. Resiliency fully unfolds when you stay in the director's chair despite any adversity you might encounter.

You become resilient by taking a position of no surrender. This is not a position of stubborn stupidity or inflexibility but one of resourcefulness and determination that you *will* find a way to achieve your goal because you will accept no other outcome. If one path does not work, you discard it and find another. Then you stick with the new one that works.

Develop the stress-resistant attitude that tough experiences are a source of valuable lessons. Purposely cultivate an internal approach to difficulties that is oriented to learning and coping rather than feeling victimized and blaming circumstances or others. If you are momentarily thrown off by setbacks, obstacles, or adversity, talk and coach yourself back to this perspective. Resolve to learn from your setback, make the necessary adjustments, and continue, knowing you are the stronger for it.

We have been talking to you about writing your own autobiography, about making choices, about directing your own movie. After all the script writing and preproduction activities, here comes that moment when, at least in the movies, they say "Lights, camera, action."

You are prepared. You know how to use the industrial-strength power tools for change. You have completed film school, and it's time to shoot your first feature. What come next are labs. Think of them as scenes from your movie. Hop in the director's chair, and get started.

real change: off track? (continued)

By completing the exercises in this chapter, Hameed, whom you read about on page 34 of Chapter 3, realized that he had not been operating from his true GPS coordinates. He had come to college with every intention of becoming a research physicist. But when he had to identify the source and inspiration for this goal, he remembered that his parents were the ones who always said he could and should go into science.

Hameed hadn't questioned his career path until his roommate asked him to help out backstage at drama department productions. Soon, enchanted by a whole new world, he couldn't learn enough about the technical aspects of lighting and stage management. His science background and experience with computers gave him skills that earned him a reputation as the go-to electronic wizard.

In Hameed's case, drifting off track didn't mean he was going in the wrong direction. He was, in fact, making a course correction and finding a new destination. At first he didn't tell his parents because he thought his new interest might just be an intellectual infatuation. He also knew stage and film production was hardly what they had in mind when they sent him to college. But each new play convinced Hameed that it was the only career he wanted to pursue.

Rather than just blurting out his plans, Hameed, ever the systematic thinker, prepared a PowerPoint presentation about careers in film and stage production, along with handouts on income projections. His parents' initial response to them was disappointment. Although it's taken some time, they have come to accept his decision. When they see Hameed's enthusiasm, his dedication, and his hard work—the very qualities they'd always nurtured in their bright and talented son—they can't help but feel proud.

SELECTED BIBLIOGRAPHY

American College Health Association. *American College Health Association National College Health Assessment Reference Group Executive Summary Fall 2006.* Baltimore: American College Health Association, 2007.

———. "American College Health Association National College Health Assessment Spring 2006 Reference Group Data Report (Abridged)." *Journal of American College Health* 55, no. 4 (January–February 2007):195–206.

Bandura, Albert. *Self-Efficacy: The Exercise of Control.* New York: Freeman, 1997.

Begley, Sharon. *Train Your Mind, Change Your Brain: How a New Science Reveals Our Extraordinary Potential to Transform Ourselves.* New York: Ballantine Books, 2007.

Benson, Herbert. *The Relaxation Response.* New York: Harper Paperbacks, 2000.

Burka, Jane, and Leonora Yuen. *Procrastination: Why You Do It, What to Do about It.* Cambridge: Perseus Books, 1983.

Christian, Kenneth W. *Your Own Worst Enemy: Breaking the Habit of Adult Underachievement.* New York: HarperCollins, 2004.

Dement, William, and Christopher Vaughan. *The Promise of Sleep: A Pioneer in Sleep Medicine Explores the Vital Connection between Health, Happiness, and a Good Night's Sleep.* New York: Dell, 2000.

Diener, Ed, R. A. Emmons, R. J. Larsen, and S. Griffin. "The Satisfaction with Life Scale." *Journal of Personality Assessment* 49 (1985):71–75.

Ellis, Albert. *Rational-Emotive Therapy.* New York: Allyn & Bacon, 1988.

Fadiman, James. *Unlimit Your Life: Setting and Getting Goals.* Berkeley: Celestial Arts, January 1990.

Goleman, Daniel. *Emotional Intelligence.* New York: Bantam, 1995.

———. *Social Intelligence.* New York: Bantam, 2006.

Gollwitzer, Peter. "Implementation Intentions: Strong Effects of Simple Plans." *American Psychologist* 54 (1999):493–503.

Haley, Jay. *Uncommon Therapy.* New York: W. W. Norton, 1993.

Monaghan, Patricia, and Eleanor Diereck. *Meditation: The Complete Guide.* Novato, CA: New World Library, 1999.

National Center on Addiction and Substance Abuse. *Wasting the Best and the Brightest: Substance Abuse at America's Colleges and Universities,* Report. New York: National Center on Addiction and Substance Abuse at Columbia University, March 2007.

Pennebaker, James. *Writing to Heal: A Guided Journal for Recovering from Trauma and Emotional Upheaval.* Oakland, CA: New Harbinger, 2004.

Prochaska, James, John Norcross, and Carlo DiClemente. *Changing for Good.* New York: William Morrow, 1992.

Rotter, Julian. "Generalized Expectancies for Internal versus External Control of Reinforcement," *Psychological Monographs* 80, whole no. 609 (1966).

Seligman, Martin. *Learned Optimism: How to Change Your Mind and Your Life.* New York: Vintage, 2006.

Taylor, Shelley, Lien Pham, Inna Rivkin, and David Armor. "Harnessing the Imagination: Mental Simulation, Self Regulation and Coping." *American Psychologist* 53 (1998):429–439.

Weil, Andrew, and Winifred Rosen. *From Chocolate to Morphine: Everything You Need to Know about Mind-Altering Drugs.* New York: Houghton Mifflin, 2004.